The
I HATE
DIETING DIET

50 WAYS TO LOSE WEIGHT AND SLIM DOWN WITHOUT
GIVING UP THE FOODS YOU LOVE OR EXERCISING

Howard VanEs, M.A.

The I Hate Dieting Diet
50 Ways to Lose Weight and Slim Down without Giving Up the
Foods You Love or Exercising

Howard VanEs, M.A.

Published by:
BooksOnHealth.net

ISBN: 978-0692490150

Disclaimer: The information and ideas presented in this book are for educational purposes only. This book is not intended to be a substitute for consulting with an appropriate health care provider. Any changes or additions to your medical care should be discussed with your physician. The author and publisher disclaim any liability arising directly or indirectly from this book.

TABLE OF CONTENTS

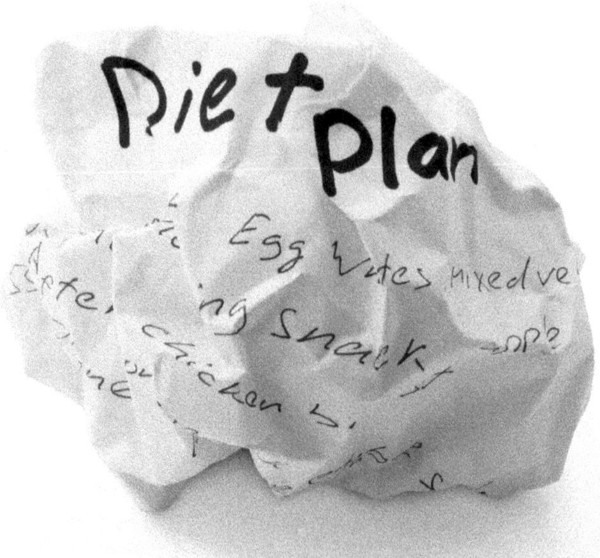
Diet Plan

INTRODUCTION
DIETS DON'T WORK!

If you ever tried one, you probably already know that you can lose weight, only to gain it all back. Most often so called "diets" end up causing frustration, guilt, and in many cases weight gain!

In fact, studies show that 95% of all diets fail. And with good reasons: they deprive you, ask you to give up whole categories of foods and nutrients, restrict your calories, and don't show you how to lose weight for the long run.

Eating shouldn't be complicated – you should be able eat the foods you love!

The *I Hate Dieting Diet* provides you with scientifically proven ways to lose weight without giving up the foods you enjoy or having to exercise. There is no shopping, no special food, no counting calories, points, meetings, or any other ridiculous behaviors that only end in frustration. We could have called it the "Dream Diet," but no dieting is needed!

As you start to incorporate the tools and ideas in the book you will see excess weight start to come off naturally and easily, and just as importantly, you'll know how to keep weight off for life. Here is a sample of some of the unique and effective methods you'll find in this book:

- **New tech ways to lose weight**

- **How massage helps with weight loss**

- **How to rev your metabolism and turn into a calorie burning furnace**

- **How and when to eat more often to lose weight**

- **The different types of fat, which is best for weight loss, and how to activate that**

- **The only supplements that have ever been shown to really help with weight loss**

- **And 44 more proven and easy ways to help you lose weight**

Now you can enjoy foods you love without feeling hungry, deprived, or frustrated with a plan that is so easy to incorporate and maintain that you can finally put an end to the vicious cycle of yoyo dieting and feel good doing it! Let's get started.

CHAPTER 1

WHY DIETS DON'T WORK

Diets simply do not work. Studies show that 95% of people who shed pounds eventually gain them back or more.[1] Unfortunately, the weight-loss market is saturated with diets that promise fast results. Often referred to as "fad diets," they are the most ineffective of all weight-loss strategies. These eating plans are usually short, extreme, and require some radical change to your diet in order to melt pounds.

As tempting as a quick fix might be, most people end up losing water weight as well as muscle that is important for burning calories. Once the "diet" is over, most dieters gain back the weight. The only problem is that now they have less muscle for burning calories, so they gain even more weight. They then go on another fad diet and start the cycle over again. Thus, we have the term *yoyo dieting*.

Here are some other reasons why most diets fail in the long run:

One Size Does Not Fit All

Most diets are formulated with a one-size-fits-all mentality and most likely will not meet your individual needs. Caloric and nutritional requirements can vary greatly from person to person, based on genetics, overall health, gender, height, lifestyle, and activity/exercise levels.

Obviously, the nutritional requirements of a 32-year-old pregnant woman are going to be different than those of a 68-year-old male heart patient. The dietary requirements of a 45-year-old sales executive are going to be different than those of a 23-year-old professional soccer player.

The best nutritional plans are ones that meet *your* specific needs!

Eliminating Food Groups

Many diets try to achieve quick weight loss by eliminating certain foods. Whether it is carbohydrates, grains, fat, or dairy, proponents of these diets claim you can shed pounds by avoiding certain food groups.

Eliminating food groups is not effective because you may be eliminating important nutrients in the process. You will also most likely end up binging on those very foods you were asked to avoid. This strategy is not only dangerous to your health but also detrimental to your weight-loss efforts. Of course, avoiding foods like refined sugars, white flour, trans fats, and salt can go a long way in helping you lose weight and improving your overall health.

Restricting Calories

While it is true that cutting back calories can help you lose weight, diets often take it too far and too fast. Reducing your calorie intake drastically can trim your body in the short term but set you up for weight "regain" in the future.

According to a study in the *New England Journal of Medicine*, people who lose weight from calorie-restrictive diets tend to be hungrier because of hormones released.[2] As your body weight decreases, the levels of leptin and ghrelin start to change.

Leptin, the hormone that regulates appetite, decreases. At the same time, levels of ghrelin—the hormone that causes hunger—increases. As a result, people start to overeat or binge to keep up with an increasing appetite and subsequently gain the weight back.

In addition to the potential of increasing your appetite, calorie-restricted diets also cause changes to our metabolism. As ironic as it sounds, studies show that your metabolism slows down as you slim down.[3] In other words, your body burns fewer calories as you lose weight from dieting.

Dieting is a vicious cycle that seems beneficial in the beginning because it causes weight loss. Your metabolism speeds up and increases your BMR (Basal Metabolic Rate) temporarily. Once you are leaner, your energy expenditure decreases because it takes fewer calories to maintain a smaller physique.

As energy expenditure decreases and metabolism slows down, it becomes easier to put the weight on again. As the pounds slowly creep back, you are likely to go on another diet and relive the process over and over again. Yoyo dieting again!

Deprivation

Deprivation is the cornerstone of dieting. Unfortunately, it triggers psychological processes that hinder weight loss and increase the chance of becoming overweight again.

One way it does this is by making "forbidden," unhealthy foods more attractive. By asking dieters to steer clear of certain foods, it only makes them more appealing. Over time, cravings for those foods intensify and eventually lead to binge eating.

A lot of weight-loss diets encourage "cheat days" when dieters can take a well-deserved break from a balanced diet. This type of thinking leads people to see unhealthy foods as rewards and eating healthy as a burden.

When eating healthy becomes something you *have* to do instead of what you *want* to do, losing weight becomes challenging. The negative emotions that dieting produces are some of the main reasons people give up on their efforts.

Inability to Maintain Results

Many diets, especially fad diets, are designed to be effective in the short term. The primary goal is to help you lose weight as quickly as possible, and not much thought is given to maintaining the new weight. Without a proper maintenance plan, many people relapse to old habits and food choices.

The diets that do include a maintenance plan that's not well thought out usually fall short. A major reason is because the maintenance plans are not very different from the original diet. More often than not, people are advised to continue following rigid eating plans and practicing unrealistic dietary habits for life.

Food Packaging

In an effort to simplify dieting, some programs have packaged food for you. Obviously this simplifies meal planning and is wonderfully convenient. The downside is that the foods are not fresh, which means they may lack optimal nutrients. These foods also often contain chemicals and preservatives that you simple don't want in your diet, as they can be toxic to your system. Moreover, diets with packaged foods don't teach you how to select foods that are going to support your health in the long run.

---

1   Sumithran, P., & Proietto, J. (2013). The defence of body weight: A physiological basis for weight regain after weight loss. *Clinical Science, 124*(4), 231-241. Retrieved from http://www.clinsci.org/cs/124/0231/cs1240231.htm

2   Sumithran, P., Luke, A., Delbridge, E., Purcell, K., Shulkes, A., Kriketos, A., & Proietto, J. (2011). Long-term persistence of hormonal adaptations to weight loss. *New England Journal of Medicine, 365*(17), 1597-1604. Retrieved from http://www.nejm.org/doi/full/10.1056/nejmoa1105816

3   Rosenbaum, M., Kissilef, H. R., Mayer, L. E. S., Hirsch, J., & Leibel, R. L. (2010). Energy intake in weight-reduced humans. *Brain Research, 1350,* 95-102. Retrieved from http://www.ncbi.nlm.nih.gov/pmc/articles/PMC2926239/

CHAPTER 2

GET COLD: TRIGGER BROWN FAT

Your body has two main types of fat: white and brown. The white fat is the one you've been working so hard to get rid of. This is because it is responsible for converting and storing extra energy as body fat.

Brown fat, on the other hand, does the exact opposite. Because it is filled with mitochondria, it helps burn the calories you eat faster and more efficiently. Triggering brown fat can boost your metabolism and turn up your body's fat-burning ability.

Activating brown fat is incredibly easy. All you have to do is expose your body to cold temperatures. Whether you are indoors or outdoors, reducing the temperature forces the fat to produce heat in order to keep you warm. Creating heat needs calories, and if they're not from food, your body will use stored body fat instead.

You can start applying this technique by turning down or switching off the heating system in your home or taking a walk on a chilly day. There is no recommendation on how much time you need to spend in the cold so listen to your body to avoid compromising your health.

The jury is still out about whether your body can make new brown fat cells. While some studies suggest it is possible, others imply otherwise. One thing for sure is that everyone has it. The amount might vary from person to person, but it is definitely there.

So next time there's a chill in the air, instead of burning energy to heat your home, burn some calories instead. As more research emerges about brown fat's ability to burn calories, this appears to be another important key to slimming down naturally.[4]

---

4   Seale, P., & Lazar, M. A. (2009). Brown fat in humans: Turning up the heat on obesity. *Diabetes, 58*(7), 1482–1484. Retrieved from http://www.ncbi. nlm.nih.gov/pmc/articles/PMC2699856/

CHAPTER 3

TECH WAYS TO LOSE WEIGHT

Technology has made life easier in so many ways, especially in health and weight loss. From social media to smart apps, more and more people are turning to "tech" to help them shed pounds. Thanks largely to the World Wide Web, anyone can turn their smartphone, tablet, or computer into a tool for weight loss. A study in the International Journal of Behavioral Nutrition and Physical Activity reported that people who use self-monitoring tools on the Web lose more weight.[5] The tools people used included food and exercise logs, electronic diaries, forums, and weight-loss programs and challenges. Here are some ways you can tap into technology:

Weight-Loss Apps

Newer, smarter apps for weight loss are emerging every year. You can download programs that help you manage daily calories, find free workouts, healthy recipes, and so much more. What's more, apps can be downloaded to your phone or "fit band" so that you can keep track of your weight loss wherever you are.

Virtual Support Groups

If you don't have access to friends or family to help keep you motivated, you can always join a virtual support group online. There are many free-to-join, online communities where people discuss weight-loss topics and share personal stories, successes, and struggles.

Sharing on Social Media

Social media networks are great platforms to share your weight goals, process, and progress with others. You can join a group or fun weight-loss challenge, post pictures of your new look, exchange tips, link to videos, and even encourage your friends to join you.

Fitness Video Games

Although they're not replacing workout DVDs any time soon, fitness video games are changing the face of exercise. Fun, interactive, and visually appealing, these games are a great way to get fit while you play.

Smart Gadgets

From wristband monitors to pedometer straps, gadgets can make melting pounds exciting and convenient. Because they are light and mobile, you can record, track info, and see progress while on the go.

5   Johnson, F., & Wardle, J. (2011). The association between weight loss and engagement with a web-based food and exercise diary in a commercial weight loss programme: A retrospective analysis. *International Journal of Behavioral Nutrition and Physical Activity, 8*(1), 83-89. Retrieved from http://www.ijbnpa.org/content/8/1/83

CHAPTER 4

SELF-HYPNOSIS

Hypnosis is a process for accessing your subconscious mind in order to change perceptions, beliefs, and habits. In traditional hypnosis, one person (the clinician) hypnotizes the other, but in self-hypnosis you are in charge of the process and decide which suggestions to feed your subconscious. Self-hypnosis has been used to treat everything from smoking to sleeping problems. But it can help you get slimmer too![6]

Positive thinking is vital to successful weight loss. If you have negative perceptions about eating healthy, lack confidence, or have trouble making important changes, you will soon run into challenges that discourage you or ruin your motivation.

Benefits of self-hypnosis include:

- **Helps you adopt a positive attitude about healthy eating habits and exercise**

- **Boosts your self-esteem and confidence**

- **Helps you to reflect on the progress you've made**

- **Shifts your focus from drawbacks to future benefits**

- **Relieves stress and fosters deep relaxation**

To practice self- hypnosis, follow these easy steps:

Preparation

Because self-hypnosis is about replacing pre-existing thoughts with new ones, you need to be prepared by jotting down things that you find most difficult about the weight-loss process. Once you know your challenges, write down opposite, positive affirmations. For example, if eating healthy food is your number one obstacle, a positive statement might be "I enjoy eating healthy food because it gives me more energy." If exercising regularly is the challenge, then an affirmation like "Exercising is fun and keeps me healthy" can do the trick.

Self-hypnosis can also be used to counter negative thoughts you have about yourself. Many people are worried that they can't lose weight, they'll gain it all back, or that being overweight makes them unattractive. To counter these perceptions, create affirmations that give you confidence, strength, and motivation. Statements such as "I will reach my goal weight," "I can keep weight off easily," or "I'm attractive no matter what I look like" are effective thoughts to reinforce.

The Hypnosis Process

Once you're clear about the objectives of hypnotizing yourself, find a quiet place where you can sit or lie down in a comfortable position. Be sure to switch off devices that might distract you and put a "Do Not Disturb" sign on your door. Close your eyes and take few long, deep breaths. Once you're relaxed, imagine yourself standing at the top of a staircase. The staircase should have 10 steps. With each step down, allow your body and mind to sink deeper into a state of complete relaxation. You're standing on the top 10th step. Go down the steps slowly, one at a time. On the 9th step, your head and face should relax. On the 8th step, your shoulders. On the 7th step, your chest and arms. On the 6th, your belly. On the 5th, your hips and buttocks. On the 4th, your thighs. On the 3rd, your calves and shins. On the 2nd, your feet and ankles should be relaxed.

Step 1 is when your body goes into a full hypnotic state. It helps to imagine a door at the bottom of the staircase. Think of this door as an entryway to your subconscious mind, the vault of your innermost thoughts.

Walk through the door into the innermost recesses of your mind. Remember that everything you say here will change your habits, perspectives, and thoughts permanently. Begin speaking the positive affirmations, stating each one clearly and confidently.

Coming out of Hypnosis

After repeating affirmations to your satisfaction, visualize yourself walking backwards until you are in front of the door once again at the bottom of the staircase. Close the door and begin walking back up the steps. With every step, you will feel your body gaining sensation and your mind easing out of hypnosis. On the last step, open your eyes and appreciate the changes you've made to your life.

---

6   Cochrane, G., & Friesen, J. (1986). Hypnotherapy in weight loss treatment. *Journal of Consulting and Clinical Psychology, 54*(4), 489-492. Retrieved from http://psycnet.apa.org/psycinfo/1986-30794-001

CHAPTER 5

SET THE TABLE RIGHT!

Before you sit down for your next meal, you may want to think twice about how you set the dining table. From the lighting to plates, how you arrange dining décor can affect how much you eat. Here are some useful tips to help you set your table for weight-loss success:

Choose Your China

The size and color of your plates play an important role in how much food you're likely to eat. Eating out of large, light-colored (or white) plates is the norm. Unfortunately, bigger plates make room for more food, which makes overeating almost inevitable.

Whether you're dining alone or with company, changing your china can make a positive difference on your waistline. Switch large plates with smaller ones to cut your portions in half. If you have white plates, replace them with blue ones. According to Roberta Anding, a dietician at the Texas Children's Hospital, the color blue can curb a raging appetite.[7] This is partly because the brain does not associate the color with food.

Reach for the Food

When dining with family and friends, avoid filling the table with food and leaving leftovers in sight. The more visible food is, the more likely you are to grab more.[8] Either fill the table with low-calorie foods or create a distance between you and food by dishing out in the kitchen or at another area.

You'll also want to sit at the head of the table because food is usually placed in the center of the dining table, thus making it difficult to reach. Creating this little obstacle can stop you from reaching for seconds or mindless picking, keeping your calorie intake in check.

Adjust Lighting

Although dim lighting can create a more relaxed atmosphere, it can lead to overeating too. Brightening the room allows you to see exactly what you're eating and how much of it.

Limit Distractions

In today's modern society, people are surrounded by all kinds of technologies. From cell phones to computers to TV sets, there are plenty of distractions. Being distracted while you eat splits your attention, making you unaware of the amount of food you're actually consuming.

Stay mindful by turning off cellphones and other devices until you're done with your meal. Eat only at the table and wait until you are finished to continue your schedule. Eating in silence and chewing your food till it is liquefied is a spiritual discipline and can satisfy your appetite with less food than normal.[9]

Watch Yourself Eat

Eating in front of a mirror might sound a little odd, but it encourages mindful eating. You can opt to sit directly in front of one or position mirrors to catch the reflection of your dining table. Watching yourself take bites of your meal can have an appetite-suppressing effect.

---

7   Myers, C. (2011). Study: Plate colors can promote weight loss. Retrieved from http://abc13.com/archive/8455455/

8   Privitera, G. J. (2013). Proximity and visibility of fruits and vegetables influence intake in a kitchen setting among college students. *Environment and Behavior, 45*(7), 876-888. Retrieved from http://eab.sagepub.com/content/45/7/876.abstract

9   Aivanhov, O. M. (1990). *The yoga of nutrition.* Frejus, France: Prosveta

CHAPTER 6

WEIGHT-LOSS SUPPLEMENTS THAT WORK

Although no one has found a miracle cure for being overweight yet, there are a few supplements that show positive results and can help your body melt those extra pounds with little effort.

Keep in mind that the FDA does not consider supplements to be medication and have put them into the category of food. With that said, it is always a good idea to consult your health care practitioner or your physician before taking any weight-loss supplements. This is especially important if you have diabetes, high blood pressure, liver disease, or other serious health conditions.

There is an overwhelming amount of supplements on the market available today. While some claim to curb your appetite, others are supposedly designed to burn calories without exercise. Unfortunately, only a few have been proven to be "possibly effective."

Green Coffee Extract

Made from green, unroasted coffee beans, it is believed to increase calorie burn and prevent carbohydrates from being absorbed in the body.[10]

This supplement contains two substances that can aid weight loss: caffeine and chlorogenic acid. Caffeine has been shown to boost metabolism temporarily. Chlorogenic acid, on the other hand, hinders the absorption of carbs that can be stored as fat.

Because green coffee supplements have high amounts of caffeine, it is possible to experience symptoms such as sleeplessness, headaches, and heart palpitations, especially if you are sensitive to caffeine. Avoid this supplement if you have any major health issues.

Whey Protein

Whey protein is usually used by active individuals to build muscle mass. However, studies indicate that it might be beneficial for weight loss too. In a 12-week clinical study, participants given a whey protein supplement lost about 6% of body fat without dieting or exercising.[11]

The substances in whey protein responsible for weight loss are leucine and, of course, protein. While leucine encourages calorie burn, protein suppresses the appetite to decrease your calorie intake.

Whether consumed as a shake or pill, whey protein is one of the safe supplements available. However, there have been reports of people experiencing nausea, headaches, fatigue, bloating, and upset stomachs.

Mango Seed Fiber

Fiber, in general, aids weight loss by improving the absorption of fats. However, some fibers are more effective than others. Mango seed fiber, also known as Irvingia Ganbonensis, was put to the test in a study involving 40 overweight participants and showed to be effective at decreasing body fat over time.[12]

Mango seed fiber is considered safe to use but can cause mild side effects such as headaches, sleeplessness, and excessive flatulence.

---

10 Thom, E. (2007). The effect of chlorogenic acid enriched coffee on glucose absorption in healthy volunteers and its effect on body mass when used long-term in overweight and obese people. *Journal of International Medical Research, 35*(6), 900-908. Retrieved from http://www.ncbi.nlm.nih.gov/pubmed/18035001

11 Frestedt, J., Zenk, J. L., Kuskowski, M. A., Ward, L. S., & Bastian, E. D. (2008). A whey-protein supplement increases fat loss and spares lean muscle in obese subjects: A randomized human clinical study. *Nutrition & Metabolism, 5*, 8. Retrieved from http://www.ncbi.nlm.nih.gov/pmc/articles/PMC2289832/

12 Ngodi, J. L.,Oben, J. E., & Minka, S. R. (2005). The effect of Irvingia gabonensis seeds on body weight and blood lipids of obese subjects in Cameroon. *Lipids Health, 4*, 12. Retrieved from http://www.ncbi.nlm.nih.gov/pmc/articles/PMC1168905/

CHAPTER 7

USE THE GLYCEMIC INDEX FOR WEIGHT LOSS

Carbohydrates were once considered the evil responsible for the obesity epidemic. As research advanced, experts discovered that it is actually the type and amount of carbs that affect our waistlines. By using the Glycemic Index, you can create a diet that keeps blood sugars stable and your figure lean.

The Glycemic Index, or GI scale, is essentially a chart of how different foods affect blood sugar levels.[13] Foods can fall into three categories: high, medium, and low GI, and actual numbers are assigned to each food with sucrose being at 100. The higher the GI of a food is, the more sugar it releases into your body. Subsequently, the lower the GI, the more stable your blood sugar will be. The GI scale also indicates how fast the carbohydrates in foods will turn into sugars. While some foods release sugars slowly, others do this at a rapid rate. This can have a very important effect on your weight and health.

Your body needs carbohydrates so it can turn them into energy for daily living. The carbs in high-GI foods are processed very quickly. As a result, too much sugar (glucose) is quickly released into your system. If your body cannot turn all of it into energy, it stores the rest as fat.

Low-GI foods, on the other hand, release sugars at a much slower pace. This gives your body time to convert them into energy, leaving no excess sugars to be converted into fat. Therefore, eating more foods with a lower GI can effectively speed up weight loss and help prevent and manage diabetes.[14]

You can use the GI scale to determine which foods you should eat most often, sometime, infrequently, or not at all. You can also mix high GI foods with low GI foods to get an overall lower GI score. You want to shoot for medium to low score.

The high end of the GI scale includes mostly:

- **Food products made from white flour and white rice**
- **Bright-colored vegetables like carrots, beets, corn, and white potatoes**
- **Most processed cereals**
- **Sweet fruits such pineapple, melons, figs, and dates**
- **Alcoholic drinks with the exception of red wine**
- **Pretzels, crackers, popcorn, candy, etc.**

- **Common medium-GI foods include:**
- **Whole grain pastas**
- **Semi-processed grains**
- **Legumes**
- **Grapes, mango, and banana**
- **Low-GI foods:**
- **Whole grains**
- **Vegetables such as lettuce, broccoli, spinach , onions, mushroom**
- **Nuts**
- **Cherries, berries, grapefruit, apples**
- **Yogurt, whole milk, some ice-cream**

You can find a more complete list of the GI values of common foods by simply searching online.

When creating your menu, it is advisable to dominate your plate with low-GI foods, have moderate amounts of medium-GI foods, and limit or avoid high-GI foods.

Even with low-GI, remember to exercise portion control. Eating too much of these foods can overload your system with unused sugars. But the right portion can boost energy levels and nutrient intake.

---

13 Foster-Powell, K., Holt, S., & Brand-Miller, J. C. (2002). International table of glycemic index and glycemic load values: 2002. *The American Journal of Clinical Nutrition, 76,* 5-56. Retrieved from http://ajcn.nutrition.org/content/76/1/5.full.pdf

14 Maki, K. C. Rains, T. M., Kaden, V. N., Raneri, K. R., & Davidson, M. H. (2007). Effects of a reduced-glycemic–load diet on body weight, body composition, and cardiovascular disease markers in overweight and obese adults. *American Society for Clinical Nutrition, 85*(3), 724-734. Retrieved from http://ajcn.nutrition.org/content/85/3/724

CHAPTER 8

THE LYMPHATIC SYSTEM AND WEIGHT LOSS

The lymphatic system is a collection of vessels in your body that carry fluids, toxins, fats, and other substances from one part of the body to another. It also transports white blood cells to and from the lymph nodes into the bones. If lymph nodes become inflamed or blocked, the effects can include bloating as well as weight gain.

In particular, fats need to get to the liver to be processed and passed out of the body. If lymph nodes swell up and fats can't reach the liver, they will be deposited throughout the body.[15] The most common places fats get deposited are in the midsection and in cells just under the skin. When fats end up under the skin, the result is cellulite.

The accumulation of toxins in the body can also cause weight gain. When lymph nodes are blocked, harmful substances can build up in the liver and hinder fat metabolism. Toxins can also cause water retention and starve cells of essential nutrients.

Lymphatic obstruction produces a range of obvious symptoms. Some of these include:

- **Increased belly fat**
- **Swelling in the legs and face**
- **Bloating**
- **Puffiness around the eyes**
- **Lack of energy**
- **Digestion problems, especially acid reflux**
- **Elevation in blood pressure and cholesterol**

Improving lymphatic movement is surprisingly easy. Here are a few ways:

Dry Brushing

Because most lymph nodes are under the skin, dry brushing can unclog these vessels and restore their function.[16] Using a bristle brush, simply brush your skin in a repetitive motion from your feet upwards. Brush in the direction of your heart for best results.

Deep Breathing

Just as blood is pumped by the heart, the lymphatic system is driven by breathing movements. The breathing practices of yoga (pranayama) can teach you to breathe deeply and stimulate the lymphatic system.

Be Active

Exercise has been shown to have stimulating effects on lymph nodes.[17] The best recommended exercise for lymphatic stimulation is rebounding: jumping on a trampoline.

Drink More H2O

Water can clear clogs and improve the flow of substances in lymph vessels. Drinking more water can also decrease water retention and help you drop a dress or pant size or two. Go for at least five to eight glasses of pure water a day. (See Chapter 14 "Get Hydrated.")

---

15   Chakraborty, S., Zawieja, S., Wang, W., Zawieja, D. C., & Muthuchamy, M. (2010). Lymphatic system acts as a vital link between metabolic syndrome and inflammation. *Annals of the New York Academy of Science, 1207*(1), E94-102. Retrieved from http://www.ncbi.nlm.nih.gov/pmc/articles/PMC2965625/

16   Mercola, J. M. (2014). Dry skin brushing: Benefits and how to. Retrieved from http://articles.mercola.com/sites/articles/archive/2014/02/24/dry-skin-brushing.aspx

17   National Lymphedema Network. (2013). NLN position paper: Exercise. Retrieved from http://www.lymphnet.org/pdfDocs/nlnexercise.pdf

CHAPTER 9

IMPROVE DIGESTION

Digestion is not an isolated process in your body. It affects other bodily processes as well, one of which is weight regulation. People with sluggish digestion are more likely to gain weight for a variety of reasons:

Intestinal Discomfort

People who experience intestinal discomfort are likely to gain weight because eating alleviates pain. This is especially true for those with stomach ulcers, irritable bowel syndrome, and acid reflux.[18] Relieving symptoms with food can cause you to eat more calories than needed.

Inflammation

Chronic digestive inflammation is another factor that can cause overeating. In an effort to heal the inflamed digestive tract, the body releases more ghrelin, an appetite-boosting hormone.[19]

Toxins in Vital Organs

The buildup of toxins in the body can cause some vital organs to malfunction. Of all organs, the liver is one of the most affected. If your liver is not functioning properly, fats that cannot be processed are sent back into the bloodstream. Liver toxicity can also increase appetite and cause abnormal fat cells to develop.[20]

Poor Absorption

For your body to burn calories efficiently, vitamins, minerals, and other nutrients in food need to be absorbed. Poor digestion hinders this absorption process. When the body senses it is being starved of nutrients, it will hold onto fat for survival.

HOW TO IMPROVE DIGESTION

Digestive issues can be caused by many factors. Some of the more common ones include poor production of enzymes, lack of good intestinal bacteria, and inadequate fiber. Fortunately, there are supplements that can help prevent and treat these problems.

Digestive Enzymes

In people with healthy digestive systems, enzymes are produced naturally by the pancreas. They help break down the food we chew into smaller components so they can be further processed into micronutrients.

Without enough digestive enzymes, you are likely to suffer from constipation, bloating, and excessive gas. If these are familiar symptoms, you can increase enzymes by eating more natural raw foods and/or fermented foods like sauerkraut and yogurt. You might also consider taking digestive enzyme supplements.

Probiotics

Probiotics are friendly bacteria needed by your intestines to process foods. These bacteria also help to keep the population of harmful bacteria low.[21] Found mostly in dairy and fermented foods, you can increase the amount of these good bacteria through diet or supplements. Foods naturally high in probiotics include yogurt, pickles, kimchi, and tempeh.

Prebiotics

Although the names sound similar, prebiotics are a type of fiber and not bacteria. Their purpose is to add strength to weak intestine walls, reduce inflammation, and keep your colon healthy. They are also available in supplements, but can be found in many fresh vegetables and fruits, including raw garlic, raw onion, raw leeks, bananas, dandelion greens, and artichokes.

---

18 El-Salhy, M., & Gundersen, D. (2015). Diet in irritable bowel syndrome. *Nutrition Journal, 14*(36). Retrieved from http://www.nutritionj.com/content/14/1/36

19 Peracchi, M., Bardella, M. T., Caprioli, F., Massironi, S., Conte, D., Valenti, L... Piodi, L. (2006). Circulating ghrelin levels in patients with inflammatory bowel disease. *Gut, 55*(3), 432–433. Retrieved from http://www.ncbi.nlm.nih.gov/pmc/articles/PMC1856072/

20 Grun, F. (2010). Obesogens. *Current Opinion in Endocrinology, Diabetes and Obesity, 17*(5), 453-459. Retrieved from http://www.ncbi.nlm.nih.gov/pubmed/20689419

21 Ringel, Y. Quigley, E. M. M., & Lin, H. C. (2012). Using probiotics in gastro-intestinal disorders. *The American Journal of Gastroenterology Supplements, 1,* 34-40. Retrieved from http://www.nature.com/ajgsup/journal/v1/n1/abs/ajgsup20127a.html

CHAPTER 10

PORTION CONTROL PLEASE!

M any people give a lot of thought to what they eat; however, it is equally important to pay attention to how much you eat, as portion control is a key factor in weight loss. Without measuring portions correctly, you can easily slip into a cycle of overeating. Here are some tips to help you size your meals.

Switch to the "New American Plate"

The American Institute of Cancer Research has devised a plan for those struggling to control portions. It is called "The New American Plate." This strategy advises filling two thirds of your plate with complex carbohydrates and a third with a protein source.[22]

By complex carbohydrates, the institute is referring to carbohydrates sourced from vegetables, fruit, and whole grains. Protein sources can be from lean meats, dairy, tofu, and other vegetarian options.

Although the New American Plate is not intended to be a diet, it is a useful guideline that can help you eat healthier for life. It combines the satiety power of protein with fiber from vegetables and whole grains for meals that are filling, low-calorie, and high in nutrients.

Weigh Your Food

Another effective method to size portions correctly is to weigh your food. Because calorie counts of foods are based on specific size servings, use a food scale to make sure you're not eating more than you think. Compare the measurements with either a food database or food label to stay within your daily limit.

Use Your Fists

If you don't have a food scale at home, you can always use everyday objects to estimate portions. The basic guidelines are:

- **Your protein source should be the size of a deck of cards**
- **Fish servings should equal the size of a checkbook**
- **Vegetable and fruit portions should be about the size of two fists**
- **Whole grains should be the size of a baseball**
- **Nuts and dried fruit should be equivalent to a golf ball or a small handful**

You can use these simple guidelines in conjunction to the New American Plate for an easy way to size portions at home.

Get It out of the Box and onto a Plate

If food comes in any form of package—whether a box or bag—serve it on a plate. Eating from the package can easily lead to overconsumption. Take out the serving you need, weigh it if necessary and transfer it to a dish.

Use Portion Planners

As the value of portion control is becoming more recognized, companies are designing lines of portion control plates and containers. These are sets of plates, food containers, and other dishware that help you size portions to help you take in fewer calories and shed weight.[23] You can find these in stores and online.

Make Eating a Challenge

An unusual yet effective method to reduce portions (and calories) is to make eating a challenge. Choosing foods that have to be peeled, sliced, or opened can help you eat less by helping you slow down. Another tip is to use utensils like chop sticks or teaspoons that only allow small bites at a time.

Split It

An effective strategy when eating at a restaurant is to split the food on your plate. As soon as food arrives on the table ask the waiter to wrap up one half to go and enjoy the other. Resist the urge to finish off the meal at home. Instead, chill it in the refrigerator and have it for lunch the next day.

---

22 American Institute for Cancer Research. (2015). The new American plate. Retrieved from http://www.aicr.org/new-american-plate/reduce_diet_new_american_plate_portion.html

23 Pedersen, S. D., Kang, J., & Kline, G. A. (2007). Portion control plate for weight loss in obese patients with type 2 diabetes mellitus. *Archives of Internal Medicine, 167*(12), 1277-1283. Retrieved from http://archinte.jamanetwork.com/article.aspx?articleid=412650

CHAPTER 11

SELF-TALK/ AFFIRMATIONS

Perhaps the biggest obstacle people face when losing weight is their own minds. If negative thinking is hindering you from achieving your weight-loss goals, positive self-talk and affirmations may be the solution to getting you back on track.

Positive self-talk or affirmations are basically the process of speaking positive statements about yourself to yourself. "I am successful" or "I have what it takes" are examples of affirmations. Affirmations can be used to change your perspective about certain things as well.

According to a study in the *Journal of the Association for Psychological Science*, positive self-talk has many advantages, including weight loss.[24] Using affirmations leads to positive thinking; thus, whenever you encounter an obstacle on your weight-loss journey, you can replace negative thoughts with proactive ones to stay focused on your goal.

A negative thought such as "Being fat is in my genes; I'll never be thinner" can be substituted with an affirmation through self-talk. If you tell yourself, "Even though I have been born with a certain set of genes, I can still successfully influence my weight and body shape," you can restore your motivation and find the strength to pursue your weight-loss goals.

Other effective affirmations for weight loss include:

- **"Eating healthy foods makes me feel vibrant and alive."**
- **"I am capable of reaching my weight-loss goals."**
- **"I take care of myself—mind and body."**
- **"My workout is the best part of my day."**
- **"I am beautiful/handsome and attractive regardless of how much I weigh."**

Begin your self-talk exercise by grabbing a pen and a sheet of paper. On one side of the sheet, write down all your fears and worries about losing weight. Describe negative emotions and thoughts that make you feel like giving up. Now, turn the sheet of paper around and replace each negative thought from the other side with a positive one. List affirmations in simple sentences that are easy to repeat. Be sure to have only positive words in your affirmations. For example, instead of saying, "I am not ugly," say, "I am beautiful."

Find a quiet place where you can speak loudly without being heard. You can even sit in front of a mirror if you prefer. Read affirmations one by one slowly, internalizing every sentence. In other words, say it and mean it.

Perform this exercise several times a day. Also try to meditate on affirmations throughout the day. Over time, you will naturally start to feel motivated, positive, and determined to reach your weight-loss goals!

---

24 Legault, L., Al-Khindi, T.L., & Inzlicht, M. (2012). Preserving integrity in the face of performance threat: Self-affirmation enhances neurophysiological responsiveness to errors. *Journal of the Association for Psychological Science, 23*(12), 1455-1460. Retrieved from http://pss.sagepub.com/content/23/12/1455

CHAPTER 12

HERBAL TEAS FOR WEIGHT LOSS

Tea has a well-earned reputation as a soothing beverage; however, research studies have shown that herbal tea benefits extend to weight loss as well. By sipping on various types of teas, you can increase your metabolism, burn more fat, conquer your appetite, and shrink your waistline.[25] And tea is a low calorie drink that tastes good too! Here are some teas that will aid your weight-loss efforts:

Mint Tea

Tea made from peppermint has an interesting effect on appetite: it reduces it. Even the act of smelling peppermint leaves can crush cravings. It can also soothe digestive issues as well.

Ginger Tea

Many people drink ginger tea to ease the symptoms of colds and flu because it contains many disease-fighting antioxidants. However, ginger tea can support weight loss by supporting your digestive system.[26] Ginger tea is known to treat constipation and other digestive ailments. By triggering digestive enzymes, food is efficiently processed into energy instead of being stored as fat. It can also amp up metabolism to increase calorie burn.

Green Tea

Of all the teas known to boost weight loss, green tea is arguably the most famous. Filled with EGCG catechins that speed up metabolism, it can help melt stored fat.[27] If you have tolerance for caffeine, you can opt for the decaf options.

Ginseng Tea

Ginseng has been used as a medicine in Asian cultures for centuries. In 2014, a group of researchers studied its effects on weight loss. Over an 8-week period, the results showed a decrease of body weight in participants who drank the tea daily.[28]

Ginseng tea also showed improvements in digestion as well. Not only does it improve the absorption of fats and nutrients, but also stimulates good bacteria in the gut essential to metabolic processes.

To get the most benefit from tea, drink three to five or more cups per day.

25   Khoithan, M., & Niemeyer, K. (2010). Using herbal remedies to maintain optimal weight. *Journal of Nurse Practitioner, 6*(2), 153-154. Retrieved from http://www.ncbi.nlm.nih.gov/pmc/articles/PMC2927017/

26   Mansour, M.S., Ni, Y.M., Roberts, A.L., Kelleman, M., Roychoudhury, A., & St-Onge, M.P.. (2012). Ginger consumption enhances the thermic effect of food and promotes feelings of satiety without affecting metabolic and hormonal parameters in overweight men: A study. *Metabolism, 61*(10), 1347-1352. Retrieved from http://www.ncbi.nlm.nih.gov/pubmed/22538118

27   Wolfram, S. (2007). Effects of green tea and EGCG on cardiovascular and metabolic health. *Journal of the American College of Nutrition, 26*(4), 373S-378S. Retrieved from http://www.ncbi.nlm.nih.gov/pubmed/17906191

28   Song, M., Kim, B., & Kim, H. (2014). Influence of Panax ginseng on obesity and gut microbiota in obese middle-aged Korean women. *Journal of Ginseng Research, 38*(2), 106-115. Retrieved from http://www.ncbi.nlm.nih.gov/pmc/articles/PMC3986624/

CHAPTER 13

EAT A BIG BREAKFAST

Breakfast has been dubbed "the most important meal of the day" for good reason. Filling up in the morning prepares your body—and metabolism—for the day ahead. The only thing better than eating breakfast is eating a bigger breakfast!

Eating a bigger breakfast and a smaller dinner might sound counterproductive, but it is surprisingly effective at speeding up weight loss. Here are some of the reasons why:

Metabolic Cycles

A study published in the popular nutritional journal Obesity shows that the metabolism goes through cycles.[29] The average body burns more energy during the day than it does in the evening. Therefore, eating more in the daytime results in calories burned more efficiently.

Tame Your Appetite

Most people wake up hungry in the mornings, as they have been fasting all night. This is why the morning meal is called break-fast. Fueling your body with a big breakfast can keep hunger satisfied for hours and help you avoid food cravings for lunch and dinner.

Make Better Food Choices

When you skip breakfast, it won't be long before your energy levels dip. When energy levels sink, most people are tempted to grab something sugary or carb-loaded. A sizeable breakfast prevents this energy depletion and puts you in the right state of mind to make healthier food choices.

It's not unusual to have a low appetite in the morning. Some people skip breakfast because they are just not hungry. If this is a problem for you, here are strategies to work up an appetite in time for your big breakfast:

Sleep

Not getting enough sleep can cause bloating in some, which mimics the feeling of being full. Make sure you get at least 7 hours of sleep to boost your appetite.

Drink Water the Night Before

Feeling queasy in the morning can kill your appetite fast. For some, it might even cause vomiting. Drinking water the night before can reduce the queasiness you feel in the morning.

Work Out in the Morning

Breaking a sweat can boost your appetite dramatically. After a workout, your body is likely to crave the energy and electrolytes lost from exercise.

Work on Your Breakfast Menu

Having the same meal for breakfast day after day can become boring. Add variety to your menu by varying your food choices. The thought of eating something new every day can give you the motivation to adopt the habit.

Break It in Two:

If you still aren't hungry after trying the above, try breaking your breakfast in two parts. Eat the first part as early as possible and then the second part an hour or so later. This will keep your energy and metabolism high and deter you from binging on sugary snacks later in the morning.

Here is an easy way to think about the size of your meals: eat breakfast like a king, lunch like a prince, and dinner like a pauper.

---

29 Jakubowicz, D., Barnea, M., Wainstein, J., & Froy, O. (2013). High caloric intake at breakfast vs. dinner differentially influences weight loss of overweight and obese women. *Obesity 21*(12), 2504 -2512. Retrieved from http://onlinelibrary.wiley.com/doi/10.1002/oby.20460/abstract

CHAPTER 14

GET HYDRATED

What is free, has zero calories, and can help you lose more weight? If you guessed water, you are right on! Water is essential to every aspect of health, including weight loss. Sipping on this life-giving liquid throughout the day can help you shed pounds faster and boost your overall well-being in a variety of ways:

Curb Your Appetite

People often confuse thirst for hunger all the time, and this is especially true if you are on a calorie-restrictive diet. By drinking water before, between, or after meals, you can avoid overeating and consequently lose weight faster.

Water is also a powerful appetite suppressant, curbing hunger while your body adjusts to eating less food. Having a glass of water whenever you feel hungry will fill your stomach and give you the same satiating feeling food gives you.

Raise Your Metabolism

Water boosts your metabolism in two ways. First, it keeps the cells in charge of the metabolic processes hydrated, which means that your body is able to break food down better and use energy from sugars more efficiently.

Secondly, your metabolism kicks into gear every time you drink water. Why? Because your body has to release enough energy to heat it. Therefore, the colder the water is, the harder your body needs to work to warm it up. Although the effect is minimal at best, it can boost weight-loss efforts over time.

Eliminate Empty Calories

Water is a great substitute for sugar-loaded beverages. By simply replacing soft drinks and juices with water, you can eliminate hundreds of empty calories. Empty calories offer little to no nutritional benefit and can widen your waistline without you being aware of it. Flavor your water with a squeeze of fresh lemon juice, a few slices of cucumber, or some fresh mint leaves.

HOW MUCH WATER DO YOU NEED TO DRINK?

Conventional wisdom says that women should drink a minimum of eight, 8-ounce glasses of water a day and men 12 glasses. If you are exercising, pregnant, or in a hot environment, you will need to drink more.[30]

---

30   Mayo Clinic. (2015). Factors that influence water needs. Retrieved from http://www.mayoclinic.org/healthy-lifestyle/nutrition-and-healthy-eating/in-depth/water/art-20044256?pg=2

CHAPTER 15

KEEP CORTISOL IN CHECK

Cortisol is a hormone that is vital to maintaining a healthy metabolism. It also affects the balance of fluids in your body. If levels of this hormone are too high or too low, you might find it difficult and even impossible to shed pounds.[31]

Cortisol levels rise when you experience adrenal fatigue, which is caused by the adrenal glands that produce cortisol coming under constant stress, and, as a result, failing to function properly. When this happens, you can gain weight very quickly, despite following a healthy lifestyle, because your body cannot metabolize foods efficiently. It also causes water retention, which can also tip the scale.

Stress is the main cause behind high cortisol.[32] The stress can be physical, psychological, or both. Major life events such as the death of a loved one, loss of a job, or divorce can spike levels. Not sleeping enough or even a hectic work schedule can affect cortisol because you're constantly under stress.

Adrenal fatigue produces a range of uncomfortable symptoms. One of the most common signs your cortisol is too high is weight gain. Other symptoms include:

- **Low energy levels, especially in the morning**
- **Poor concentration**
- **Increased abdominal fat**
- **Erratic blood sugar levels**
- **Longer recovery periods after infections, injuries, and medical procedures**
- **Problems sleeping**
- **Irregular blood pressure**
- **Cravings for high-sugar or high-sodium foods**
- **Sluggish digestion and other gastrointestinal issues**

HOW DO YOU LOWER CORTISOL?

There are a few strategies you can use lower cortisol or prevent it from rising. Incorporate these into your lifestyle to speed up weight loss:

De-stress

People often underestimate the effects of stress on the body. Stress not only strains adrenal glands, but can also lead to other health problems. To manage stress, set aside time every day to relax. Meditate to clear your mind, take naps, read a book, practice breathing techniques, take a bath, go for a walk, or do other activities that calm you.

Sleep More

People who sleep less than 7 hours a day have been reported to have higher cortisol levels.[33] Therefore, you want to aim for 7-9 hours of shuteye every day. If you have sleeping problems, avoid consuming caffeine products past noon and try to relax a few hours before bed. Turn off the computer and TV. Turn on some relaxing music, take a warm bath, and/or enjoy a cup of chamomile tea. If you still have trouble sleeping, you may want to check out my book: Insomnia: How Can I Get to Sleep? Your Guide to Overcoming Insomnia, Sleeplessness, and Getting a Good Night Sleep.

Get a Massage

Enjoying a massage can lower cortisol and increase hormones that reduce feelings of depression. In addition, massage therapy can improve circulation to reduce the appearance of stubborn cellulite. (See the chapter on Massage and Weight Loss.)

---

31 Anagnostis, P., Athyros, V. G., Tziomalos, K., Karagiannis, A., & Mikhailidis, D. P. (2009). The pathogenetic role of cortisol in the metabolic syndrome: A hypothesis. *The Journal of Clinical Endocrinology and Metabolism* *94*(8), 2692-2701. Retrieved from http://press.endocrine.org/doi/abs/10.1210/jc.2009-0370

32 Kirschbaum, C., Prussner, J. C., Stone, A. A., Federenko, I., Gaab, J., Lintz, D.... Hellhammer, D. H. (1995). Persistent high cortisol responses to repeated psychological stress in a subpopulation of healthy men. *Psychosomatic Medicine, 57*(5), 468-474. Retrieved from http://journals.lww.com/psychosomaticmedicine/Abstract/1995/09000/Persistent_High_Cortisol_Responses_to_Repeated.9.aspx

33 Rodenbeck, A., & Hajak, G. (2001). Neuroendocrine dysregulation in primary insomnia. *Europe Pubmed Central, 157*(11), S57-61. Retrieved from http://europepmc.org/abstract/med/11924040

CHAPTER 16

LIVER CLEANSE FOR WEIGHT LOSS

One of the most important tasks of a liver is to break down fats and make sure they leave the body. If fats cannot be metabolized properly, they have no other option but to return to your bloodstream. When this happens, fat is deposited in different parts of your body. To put it plainly, you gain weight.

Another important function of the liver is filtering out toxins and extra fluids. Normally, harmful substances pass through the liver and exit with urine or fecal matter. If your liver is not working optimally, these toxins can build up and eventually lead to water retention, also known as "water weight."

Getting rid of toxic buildup can restore the organ's function and improve your potential to lose weight. In addition to improving metabolism, a liver cleanse can also improves digestion, blood sugar, blood pressure, and many other aspects of health.

Cleansing the liver is a fairly simple process, as there are certain foods and herbs that naturally contain cleansing properties.

Beet Juice

Beet juice is particularly helpful for clearing liver toxins, as it contains a substance called betaine, which is believed to have a cleansing effect.[34] If beet juice doesn't sound appetizing, you can eat fresh beets alone or as part of a meal.

Olive Oil

Olive oil seems like an unlikely solution because it contains fat; however, it is the kind of fat that can help absorb harmful toxins that plague the liver. You'll want to use organic, extra virgin olive oil, which is the purest.

Green Vegetables

Green vegetables like spinach and cabbage can have detoxifying effects on the liver. Although it's not quite clear what the cleansing agent is in these veggies, some experts believe it is the chlorophyll, which helps remove toxins from the body.

Turmeric

To prevent toxins from overloading the liver, consider adding turmeric to your spice rack. The curcumin in turmeric can promote the production of liver enzymes and may treat liver disease.[35] Turmeric is also known for its anti-inflammatory properties

Milk Thistle (Silybum Marianum)

Milk Thistle is a herb that is well known for its ability to support the liver. It contains a compound called silymarin which protects the liver cell damage and, at the same time, stimulates liver cell regeneration. Silymarin also helps to prevent the loss of glutathione, an important nutrient for liver detoxification.

Note: When it comes to cleansing, it is best to be gentle with your body. Avoid the miracle "3-day cleanse" or other cleanses that are more extreme. Eating and juicing with the above foods, spices, and herbs will safely help you over the long term. And it is always a good idea to consult with a health care practitioner to be sure you are doing the right thing for your body.

---

34 Kathirvel, E., Morgan, K., Nandgiri, G., Sandoval, B. C., Caudill, M. A., Bottiglieri, T., … Morgan, T. R. (2010). Betaine improves nonalcoholic fatty liver and associated hepatic insulin resistance: A potential mechanism for hepatoprotection by betaine. *American Journal of Physiology - Gastrointestinal and Liver Physiology, 299*(5), G1068–G1077. Retrieved from http://www.ncbi.nlm.nih.gov/pmc/articles/PMC2993168/

35 O'Cornell, M. A., & Rushworth, S. A. (2008). Curcumin: Potential for hepatic fibrosis therapy. *British Journal of Pharmacology, 153*(3), 403-405. Retrieved from http://www.ncbi.nlm.nih.gov/pmc/articles/PMC2241785/

CHAPTER 17

ESSENTIALS OILS FOR WEIGHT LOSS

Perhaps the oldest form of health care, essential oils have been used by cultures around the world for their therapeutic and healing qualities for thousands of years. When it comes to weight loss, they provide a host of benefits such as reducing food cravings and hunger, stabilizing blood sugar, improving mood , and enhancing metabolic performance. What's more, they smell and taste great too! Below is a list of common essential oils that can help you on your weight-loss journey.

Note: When using essential oils, be sure to research the source well, as all oils are not created equal. Minimally, you'll want to look for therapeutic grade, organic oils that are tested for purity from reputable vendors. You also want 100% oils, anything else has been diluted.

Essential oils are very strong, so be sure to use just one or two drops to begin with to see how they affect you if you haven't used them before.

Cinnamon Oil

Cinnamon oil can boost your weight-loss efforts, as it contains substances that decrease the amount of sugar in the bloodstream after meals.[36] Having less glucose in your system means fewer sugars for your body to turn into fat.

This essential oil has also been shown to decrease carbohydrate absorption, which not only disturbs blood sugar levels but also is associated with obesity.

You can add cinnamon oil to your daily routine by mixing a few drops with water and a dash of honey. This drink is best taken first thing in the morning and before bedtime. You can also add the oil to food or inhale the oil to decrease your appetite before meals.

Lemon Oil

Lemon oil can help you lose extra pounds by normalizing your digestive system. Known for its cleansing effect, it can help clear your stomach of undigested foods, relieving constipation and other conditions. With your digestive system at its best, your body is more efficient at burning calories. Lemon oil is also very uplifting and will improve your mood and focus.

You can combine a couple of lemon oil drops with water to make a refreshing drink or add to olive oil to make a delicious salad dressing. Diffusing it brings a wonderful fresh scent to your home or office.

Another way to use it is to soak a cotton ball with the oil and applying it directly on your skin to get rid of toxins in the cells.

Ginger Oil

Ginger oil is a multipurpose treatment for anything from the sniffles to an upset stomach. Its weight-loss benefits include the ability to increase fat burn, decrease the appearance of cellulite, and encourage fat absorption.[37]

Ginger oil makes a great bath solution to soak away aches and pains. As a topical treatment, you can apply a few drops to areas where you have cellulite and massage the skin in a circular motion. Diffuse to improve energy.

Grapefruit Oil

Using grapefruit oil can help decrease your weight in several ways. First, it helps to eliminate from your lymphatic system toxins that can obstruct fat-burning organs and cause weight gain.

Second, it promotes a process called lipid perox-idation, where types of fat are destroyed in order to lower bad cholesterol.[38] Lastly, grapefruit oil contains antioxidants, such as vitamin C, that break down toxins to prevent water retention and bloating.

You can combine grapefruit oil with ginger or lemon to add to your bath. Soak in the water for 20-30 minutes to eliminate toxins from cells. Like other oils, you can mix it with normal water to make a cleansing drink or massage it into your skin. You can also diffuse it as well for a wonderful fresh scent.

Peppermint Oil

Peppermint oil has a very distinctive and soothing aroma. In addition to its calming effect, the oil can also restrain your cravings so you can manage calories.[39] Inhaling or drinking peppermint oil can create the feeling of fullness. It also improves breathing for better workouts.

This aromatic oil's calming quality can help relieve everyday stress. Prolonged stress can burden your thyroid and pituitary glands, causing metabolism to slow down.

You can add it to your bath in the mornings, diffuse it, add a drop to your drinking water, or soak a cotton ball to fill your car with the scent. You can also simply put a drop on your hand, rub your hands together, and then cup them over your nose, taking a few deep breaths—a great pick me up! If you are experiencing digestive issues, you can also rub a little directly on your stomach.

---

36   Shihabudeen, M. S., Hansi, P. D., & Thirumurugan, K. (2011). Cinnamon extract inhibits a-glucosidase activity and dampens postprandial glucose excursion in diabetic rats. *Nutrition & Metabolism, 8*(1), 46. Retrieved from http://www.ncbi.nlm.nih.gov/pubmed/21711570

37   Westerterp-Platenga, M.. Diepvensa, K., Joosena, A. M. C. P., Bérubé-Parentc, S., & Tremblayc, A. (2006). Metabolic effects of spices, teas and caffeine. *Physiology and Behavior, 89*(1), 85-91. Retrieved from http://www.sciencedirect.com/science/article/pii/S0031938406000540

38   Gorinstein, S., Leontowicz, H., Leontowicz, M., Krzeminski, R., Gralak, M., Delgado-Licon, E.... Trakhtenberg, S. (2005). Changes in plasma lipid and antioxidant activity in rats as a result of naringin and red grapefruit supplementation. *Journal of Agricultural Food Chemistry, 53*(8), 3223-3228. Retrieved from http://pubs.acs.org/doi/abs/10.1021/jf058014h

39   Reed, J. A., Almeida, J., Wershing, B., & Raudenbush, B. (2008). Effects of peppermint scent on appetite control and calorie intake. *Appetite, 51*(2), 393.

CHAPTER 18

EAT MORE FIBER

Filling and delicious, fiber-rich foods can curb your appetite, control blood sugar, trim your waistline naturally, improve digestion, and contribute to overall good health. And the American Society for Nutritional Sciences agrees, suggesting that fiber is a very important key to staying slim and avoiding obesity, and should be included regularly in the diet.[40]

Unlike other food substances, fiber does not get broken down or absorbed in the body. It retains its composition from ingestion until it is excreted. It is this ability to stay intact that makes it useful. Instead of being absorbed into the bloodstream, fiber helps to move all the other food substances along the digestive tract. It also affects the speed at which foods move into and out of your stomach.

There are two basic types of fiber: one is soluble and the other insoluble. Soluble fiber dissolves in liquids and forms a gel that binds itself to other food substances. Insoluble fiber, on the other hand, does not dissolve and maintains its structure throughout the digestion process.

Appetite is one of the most important factors in weight loss. What and how much you eat helps determine whether you lose, gain, or maintain weight. Fiber can help manage appetite successfully by delaying hunger[41] and limiting the absorption of fats.

Because of its ability to attach to other foods, soluble fiber decelerates digestion. By slowing down digestion, it helps you stay full and feel hungry less often. This way, you can eat fewer calories and lose weight with fewer hunger pangs.

Another way fiber aids weight loss is through absorption. Although the effect is minimal, soluble fiber can prevent a small portion of fats and sugars from being absorbed in the bloodstream.

Insoluble fiber, on the other hand, is known to expand in the gut—taking up more space in the stomach. This means you can fill up on less food. Another benefit of this type of fiber is that its food sources are naturally low in calories.

In addition to weight loss, fiber has a list of other benefits too. It supports healthy digestion by regulating the frequency of bowel movements, preventing constipation, and firming up loose stools. Fiber is also known to reduce cholesterol in people at risk of heart disease, and to help diabetics manage blood sugar levels.

HOW DO YOU UP FIBER INTAKE?

Increasing your fiber intake is easy. You just need to include fresh, whole foods in your menu. Although different foods are rich in certain types of fiber, you'll want to focus on eating a combination of both soluble and insoluble.

Sources of soluble fiber include:

- **Whole grains (especially barley and oat bran)**
- **Legumes**
- **Green vegetables**
- **Citrus fruits**
- **Flaxseeds**
- **Sources of insoluble fiber include:**
- **Whole grains (especially wheat bran)**
- **Beans**
- **Skins of most fruits**
- **Green vegetables**
- **Popcorn (without butter)**

---

40 Burton-Freeman, B. (2000). Dietary fiber and energy regulation. *Journal of Nutrition, 130*(2), 272S-275S. Retrieved from http://jn.nutrition.org/content/130/2/272S.full

41 Willis, H. J. (2009). Greater satiety response with resistant starch and corn bran in human subjects. *Nutrition Research, 29*(2), 100-105. Retrieved from http://www.nrjournal.com/article/S0271-5317(09)00015-3/abstract

CHAPTER 19

MEDITATE ON IT!

T he practice of meditation has been around thousands of years and originally came about as a spiritual practice, but its benefits extend beyond that, including weight loss. Here are some ways that mediation can you help you achieve your weight-loss goals:

Increase Body Awareness

In today's world, everybody is always in a rush. Busy work schedules and hectic lifestyles have led people to eat mindlessly. From having breakfast on the go to eating dinner in front of the television, body awareness has diminished.

Lack of body awareness can cause you to miss natural cues that prevent weight gain. It becomes difficult to tell when you're full, when you're thirsty instead of hungry, and how certain foods affect your health. Meditation can restore the mind-body connection and help you become aware of your body's real needs.[42] You will also become more aware of your behaviors around food and why you select them.

Reduce Stress

Emotional and physical stress can hinder weight loss in a number of ways. One way it does this is by stressing your adrenal glands. Adrenal glands are an important component of your metabolism. They secrete a hormone called cortisol. When you're stressed, cortisol increases, slows down metabolism, and causes rapid weight gain.[43]

Increased cortisol levels can also affect your pituitary gland, another organ responsible for metabolizing calories. When the pituitary gland is disturbed, it can release inadequate amounts of thyroid hormone and cause metabolism to become sluggish. Meditation is a great antidote to stress and returns the mind-body back to balance.

Let Go of Negative Thoughts

During the process of losing weight, it is easy to experience negative thoughts and emotions. This is often the case when you run into an obstacle that impedes your progress. Meditation encourages you to let go of negative thoughts and look at them from a distance so you can gain a better perspective and clarity. Meditation will help you connect with a deeper place inside yourself that is wise, peaceful, and balanced. You can also use it to focus on positive thoughts and the benefits of achieving your weight-loss goals. Find time to meditate daily to keep yourself motivated and confident.

HOW TO MEDITATE:

There are many ways to meditate and perhaps the simplest method is to simply follow your breath. Start by sitting in a comfortably seated position with your eyes closed. Notice how your breath enters your body and how it leaves. Let the breath do its thing. There is no need to control it; just watch it. It is natural to have thoughts that interrupt this process—when you do, just bring your awareness back to the breath. You may have to do this several times. Plan on 10 to 20 minutes each time you meditate. For more information on meditation and the many ways you can practice, check out my book *Meditation, the Gift Inside.*

---

42 Daubenmier, J. J. (2005). The relationship of yoga, body awareness, and body responsiveness to self-objectification and disordered eating. *Psychology of Women Quarterly, 29*, 207-219. Retrieved from http://chc.ucsf.edu/pdf/2005_article_Daubenmier%20PWQ.pdf
43 Wilson, J. L. (2013). Clinical perspective on stress, cortisol and adrenal fatigue. *Advances in Integrative Medicine, 1*(2), 93-96. Retrieved from http://www.aimedjournal.com/article/S2212-9626%2814%2900005-4/abstract

CHAPTER 20

SNOOZE TO GET SLIM

S leep deprivation is a major cause of obesity, and the hours of sleep you don't get each night can directly affect your weight. Several research studies confirm this, including one published by the National Center for Biotechnology Information, which showed that sleep-deprived individuals gain more weight than those who sleep 7-9 hours per night.[44] Here are some of the reasons why:

Low Energy Levels Lead to Higher Carb Intake

When tiredness settles in, it is only natural to reach out for food as an energy source. Unfortunately, many people end up choosing carb-loaded, sugary foods to get an instant boost. If this happens regularly, weight gain is inevitable. Additionally, if your energy levels are low, the last thing you will want to do is exercise or do other activity. A sedentary lifestyle dramatically increases the risk of weight gain over time.

Lack of Sleep Stirs up Your Appetite

In addition to making the wrong food choices, sleepless dieters tend to have bigger appetites. This is because staying awake requires more energy. The longer you fight off the instinct to sleep, the more food your body needs to stay awake. This can lead to late night snacking and, therefore, more calories per day.

Another way not getting enough sleep adds to your appetite is by decreasing leptin levels. Leptin is the hormone that informs your brain you are full. If leptin levels are low, you will have a harder time telling if you are satiated or not, and this leads to overeating. As mentioned earlier in this book, studies also show that ghrelin, a hormone that increases hunger, is increased when you don't have enough sleep.

Sleep Deprivation Decreases Insulin Sensitivity

Insulin sensitivity refers to how well your fat cells use insulin to regulate blood sugar. A lack of sleep will decrease this sensitivity and can cause your fat cells to malfunction, allowing fats to circulate in your bloodstream. This phenomenon has been associated with the onset of obesity and other health problems.

If you have trouble sleeping, try going to sleep and waking at the same time every day until you are in a new sleeping pattern. This will reset your sleep/wake cycle. Also, be sure to ditch the coffee in the afternoon and turn off the TV and computer 1-2 hours before bedtime. Remember you want to get 7-9 hours of sleep.

If you are suffering from insomnia, please check out my book Insomnia: How Can I Get to Sleep?, available on Amazon and at www.booksonhealth.net

---

44 Patel, S. R. (2008). Short sleep duration and weight gain: A systematic review. *Obesity, 16*(3), 643-653. Retrieved from http://www.ncbi.nlm.nih.gov/pubmed/?term=%22Obesity+(Silver+Spring)%22%5Bjour%5D+Short+sleep+duration+and+weight+gain%3A+a+systematic+review

CHAPTER 21

REV UP YOUR METABOLISM

Your metabolism is an intricate web of processes that controls your weight by converting the food and drink you consume into energy. Your activity levels, stress levels, age, health, body composition, and gender all affect your metabolism. Also affecting your metabolism is the rate at which your body burns calories and processes food. Take in too many calories, and you will gain weight; take in fewer than you need, and you will lose weight. Here are a few ways to increase the rate at which you burn calories throughout the day so you can accelerate your body's fat-burning power.

Start Your Day Right

Every morning is an opportunity to prepare your body for maximum calorie burned. Begin each day with a cup of coffee or green tea to rev up your metabolism. Studies show that caffeine[45] and certain substances in herbal teas can help you melt fat for hours. If you are sensitive to caffeine, it is best to avoid this weight-loss strategy.

Spice up Your Menu

From your first meal of the day to the last, adding spice to your meals can boost your metabolism. In particular, spices made from hot peppers contain capsaicin, which has been shown to heat up the body to melt fat naturally.[46] Adding a little cayenne pepper to your meals can reduce your dress or pant size over time.

Other herbs and spices to try are turmeric, cinnamon, and peppermint. All these are available in powdered form and as essential oils. They can help suppress cravings for unhealthy foods and keep your calorie intake low.

Eat Something Different

It is easy to fall into the pattern of eating the same meals every day. Many people repeat meals to make sure they consume the same amount of calories daily. While this might help you manage calories, it can potentially slow down metabolism.

To keep your metabolism up, vary your meals and calories. Try new recipes as often as you can. If you eat 1,500 calories one day, eat 1,400 the next day and 1,700 the next. This will keep your metabolism guessing and working efficiently. You can also experiment with adjusting the ratio of protein, carbohydrates, and fats you take in daily

Snack on Gum

Keeping your mouth busy chewing gum can help reduce food cravings and delay hunger. The flavor of gum also satisfies your appetite for sweet treats, especially peppermint gum.

To protect your waistline and your teeth, opt for sugar-free gum. It contains far less sugar, if any, making it low in calories.

Fidget More

Activity burns calories, whether you're tapping your feet to music or braiding your hair. Fidgeting can increase the amount of calories you burn per minute. Avoid standing still or sitting in one position for a long time, as this could decrease your resting metabolic rate.

Get on Your Feet

One easy way to keep your metabolism up and running is to get on your feet. Because people tend to spend long hours sitting at work, make an effort to stand up and burn more calories during the day.

By simply walking around the office, getting a stand-up desk, or standing up every time the phone rings, you can torch excess fat. Working standing up can burn up to 129 calories per hour compared to 72 calories sitting down. While standing, move around to optimize results.

45 Dulloo, A. G., Geissler, C. A., Horton, T., Collins, A., & Miller, D. S. (1989). Normal caffeine consumption: Influence on thermogenesis and daily energy expenditure in lean and postobese human volunteers. *American Journal of Clinical Nutrition, 49*(1), 44-50. Retrieved from http://ajcn.nutrition.org/content/49/1/44.long

46 Janssens, P. H. R., Hursel, R., Martens, E. A. P., & Westerterp-Plantenga, M. S. (2013). Acute effects of capsaicin on energy expenditure and fat oxidation in negative energy balance. *PLoS One, 8*(7), e67786. Retrieved from http://www.ncbi.nlm.nih.gov/pmc/articles/PMC3699483/

CHAPTER 22

SIZE DOES MATTER – PLATE SIZE THAT IS!

How you perceive the amount of food you eat can help you eat less and lose weight effortlessly. This is based on a scientific concept called the Delboeuf Illusion. Studies published in the American Psychological Association show that larger plates appear to contain less food but actually carry more.[47] Small plates, on the other hand, carry less food but appear fuller. By eating from small plates, your mind will believe you're eating more while you are actually cutting back.

It is not just the size of your dishware that matters. The shape matters also. Flat plates are preferred over bowls because they hold less food in general.

What you serve on the plates is equally important. A large, fatty burger on a small plate still carries hundreds of bad calories.

In order to take advantage of this weight-loss technique, you need to follow a balanced diet. The focus of your menu should be on adding nutrient-dense foods and limiting calorie-dense products. You'll also want to avoid seconds. If you still feel hungry after your meal, opt for a glass of water to curb your appetite.

Lastly, ease into it. Like any lifestyle change, it is advisable to take your time and let your body adjust. Try decreasing the size of your dishware gradually or transitioning one meal at a time.

---

47   Wansink, B., & van Ittersum, K. (2013). Portion size me: Plate-size induced consumption norms and win-win solutions for reducing food intake and waste. *Journal of Experimental Psychology: Applied, 19*(4), 320-332. Retrieved from http://psycnet.apa.org/journals/xap/19/4/320/

CHAPTER 23

MASSAGE AND WEIGHT LOSS

For many people, having a massage is a relaxing, feel-good activity. However, there are important advantages for weight loss, including boosting fat metabolism and draining toxins from the body.[48]

Enhance Circulation and Nutrient Absorption

Just beneath your skin are hundreds upon hundreds of lymph vessels and nodes. These vessels transport everything from nutrients to toxins. If your circulation is poor, the substances lymph vessels carry can end up in the wrong place and cause you to pack on unnecessary pounds.

Cellulite, for instance, is a result of lymph nodes failing to absorb lipids (fats) from your blood. Belly fat can increase if your lymphatic system cannot get rid of toxins and bloating from poor secretion of excess fluids.

Lymph vessels and nodes are also responsible for transporting and delivering various nutrients to cells. Stimulating lymph vessels can ensure your tissues and vital organs receive the resources they need. Proper nutrient absorption can improve weight loss by making sure your cells don't starve. When cells don't receive nutrients, your energy stores can become depleted and cause you to look for alternative sources of fuel. More often than not, people turn to sweet, high-calorie drinks and caffeine for a quick boost.

A simple massage can normalize the function of your lymphatic system and blood vessels by improving circulation.

Prevent Bloating

Bloating can occur if the excess fluids in your body are not eliminated or neutralized. When these fluids accumulate, you can become bloated and go up a dress or pant size. Massages help move these fluids along and flush them from your system.

Beat Stress and Feel Good

Stress can be associated with a rise in cortisol, which is a hormone that can slow down the metabolism of fats. Not dealing with stress can also cause your thyroid gland, another metabolism-regulating organ, to malfunction.

Massages are great at alleviating physical stress caused by busy, strenuous lifestyles. Eliminating both psychological and physical stress can help your body function at its best.

One of the benefits of massage therapy is the release of "happiness hormones." Serotonin and dopamine are two hormones that have been shown to reduce depression.[49] So if you're feeling discouraged about weight loss or just running low on confidence, a massage might just be what you need.

Normalize Digestion

Some digestive problems like intestinal inflammation can cause weight gain. A therapeutic massage can trigger peristalsis to alleviate constipation and stimulate other digestive organs. It can also strengthen intestines to absorb fats better.[50]

Expel Toxins

Toxins are everywhere: in processed food, cleaning products, cosmetics, water, and even in the air we breathe. Fortunately, the liver can expel them naturally in most cases, provided circulation is working properly. If your circulatory system is not functioning at its best, these toxins can gather in the liver, resulting in extra pounds and/or illness.

Getting a massage helps eliminate toxins by improving circulation, which aids in the removal of toxins. As a result, the liver burns fat more efficiently, helping you to get leaner naturally.

---

48   Von der Weid, P. Y., & Rainey, K. J. (2010). Review article: Lymphatic system and associated adipose tissue in the development of inflammatory bowel disease. *Alimentary Pharmacology and Therapeutics, 32*(6), 697-711. Retrieved from http://onlinelibrary.wiley.com/doi/10.1111/j.1365-2036.2010.04407.x/full

49   Field, T., Hernandez-Reif, M., Diego, M., Schanberg, S., & Kuhn, C. (2005). Cortisol decreases and serotonin and dopamine increase following massage therapy. *International Journal of Neuroscience, 115*(10), 1397-1413. Retrieved from http://informahealthcare.com/doi/abs/10.1080/00207450590956459

50   Ernst, E. (1999). Abdominal massage therapy for chronic constipation: A systematic review of controlled clinical trials. *Research in Complimentary Medicine, 6,* 149-151. Retrieved from http://www.karger.com/Article/Abstract/21240

CHAPTER 24

VISUALIZE IT!

Most of us use visualization more often than we realize. The simple act of imagining your healthier self or posting a picture on the wall are all visualization techniques. This is the same process that world-class athletes use when preparing to win a major competition.

Visualization is a powerful motivating technique that can help you overcome challenges in your weight-loss journey by helping you awaken positive emotions and encouraging you to keep going. Another advantage of visualization is that it nurtures your self-esteem. It is normal to be critical of yourself when trying to lose weight. Focusing on progress made or what you can achieve can increase confidence, drive, and self-compassion.

Although everyone has a unique way of visualizing, here are variety of ways to try:

Future Thinking

This visualization technique is about seeing yourself in the future after you have accomplished your weight-loss goals.[51] It could be anything from seeing yourself wearing a smaller dress or pant size to receiving a compliment from a loved one. These visualizations need to be detailed to have a positive impact and should be reviewed many times throughout the day, especially in the morning when you awaken and before you go to sleep.

Creating a Symbol

Another way to use visualization is by creating a symbol of your success or a symbol of some internal resource that will help you achieve your goals. To create a symbol, simply close your eyes and take a few deep breaths. Then let an image come to mind that represents your future success with weight loss or an internal resource. To make this even more powerful, find a picture of your symbol or draw it and then put it someplace in your home and/or office where you will see it often.

Timelining

Timelining is a technique that documents or records your weight-loss journey. You can record your experience and progress by using pictures of yourself at various stages. Some prefer adding a journal, video diary, and even medical reports.[52]

51 De Vito, S., Gamboz, N., & Brandimonte, M. A. (2012). What differentiates episodic future thinking from complex scene imagery? *Conscious Cognition, 21*(2), 813-823. Retrieved from http://www.ncbi.nlm.nih.gov/pubmed/22342534

52 Sheridan, J., Chamberlain, K., & Dupuis, A. (2011). *Sage Journals, 11*(5), 552-569. Retrieved from http://qrj.sagepub.com/content/11/5/552.abstract

CHAPTER 25

STRATEGIES FOR EATING AT RESTAURANTS

Whether it be a work-related event, a social gathering, or a matter of convenience, we all find ourselves eating out at restaurants from time to time. While it's true that there are a lot of temptations at restaurants and people tend to overeat when visiting them, there are many strategies you can use to be in control and not blow your diet. Here are few strategies that will help:

Choose a Restaurant Thoughtfully

Start by choosing a restaurant that serves healthier options. Avoid buffets and restaurants that encourage platters and supersized meals. Not surprisingly, studies show that people tend to eat more at buffets than in any other type of restaurant setting.[53]

Browse the menu for low-calorie options before leaving the house. Many restaurants have menus online, and others even include the calorie count of dishes as well.

Order Healthy

Make sure you don't show up ravenous! When you arrive at the restaurant, avoid having bread and other starters. Instead, you can ask for a glass of water, which can help control your appetite. You can even ask your server to not bring bread to the table. For your main meal, order a dish that is rich in protein. High-protein meals have more satiating power and can help you resist the urge to overeat.[54]

To lower calories, ask for your food to be grilled, baked, steamed, or poached instead of fried. If the dish comes with sauces or sides, have them served on separate plates. Also, be mindful of the beverage you choose. Stick with healthy options like water, red wine, and unsweetened drinks like ice tea or herbal tea.

Reduce Your Portion

Portion size is arguably the biggest challenge with eating out. Because restaurants tend to serve supersized portions, reduce yours by sharing a meal with a friend. Another great strategy is to divide the meal. Eat half at the restaurants and take the other half home. Ask for a take home container when you place your food order.

Be Cautious with Sides and Desserts

Most dishes come with sides. The options are usually fries, breads, and vegetables. To stay within your calorie budget, opt for one with the least calories or don't order one at all. It is best to avoid sides that have already been seasoned or dressed, as these normally contain hidden fats and sugars.

If you can, skip dessert and have another glass of water. If you're still hungry, look through the menu for low-calorie treats. The best desserts are those that have plenty of fresh fruit and low-fat dairy. Avoid sugary, buttery, or creamy options to avoid empty calories.

---

53   Wansink, B., & Payne, C. R. (2012). Eating behavior and obesity at Chinese buffets. *Obesity, 16*(8), 1957-1960. Retrieved from http://onlinelibrary.wiley.com/doi/10.1038/oby.2008.286/full

54   Astrup, A. (2005). The satiating power of protein – A key to obesity prevention? *The American Journal of Clinical Nutrition, 82*(1). Retrieved from http://ajcn.nutrition.org/content/82/1/1.full%3E

CHAPTER 26

TEST YOUR THYROID

If you are doing everything you can to lose weight but you can't seem to take off those extra pounds, you might have a thyroid problem. Your metabolism is a complex network of processes that are governed mostly by the thyroid gland. In order for your body to burn food for energy, this gland needs to release healthy amounts of hormone. When it doesn't, a wide range of symptoms can occur, one of which is weight gain.[55]

Causes of thyroid problems include autoimmune diseases, medications, congenital defects, pregnancy, nutritional deficiencies, and a pituitary gland that is damaged and failing to stimulate thyroid. Another way you can develop hyperthyroidism is through medical procedures designed to treat the very condition. It is not uncommon for doctors to surgically remove part of a gland as part of treatment, which reduces the amount of hormone produced.

The most common ways to treat thyroid disorders is through medications, radiation therapy, and surgery. However, there are natural treatments and over-the-counter supplements that may be helpful too:

Modify Your Menu

Adding more protein and healthy fats to your diet can improve thyroid function. Protein can help carry thyroid hormones to cells to stabilize metabolism. Healthy fats can help restore hormonal balance.

Another helpful change you can make to your menu is to reduce simple carbohydrates. Simple carbs and sugars are found mostly in processed foods. Decreasing the consumption of baked goods and sugar-loaded snacks can improve thyroid gland performance.

Get Enough Nutrients

Nutrients, especially minerals, have a profound effect on how well your thyroid functions. Aim to meet the recommended intake of copper, iodine, selenium, and zinc. You can up your mineral intake by either eating nutrient-rich foods or taking vitamin supplements. Not all supplements are created equal and some do more harm than good. Be sure to consult a nutritional expert or naturopath before starting a regimen of vitamin supplements.

Improve Digestion

Scientific research has discovered a link between thyroid function and digestion.[56] Increasing the population of healthy intestinal bacteria can relieve some symptoms of hyperthyroidism. If you are prone to digestive problems, consider taking probiotics, prebiotics, and digestive enzymes.

Get Physical

Exercising while suffering from a thyroid disorder might seem pointless, but it can actually help stimulate hormone production. You don't need to jump right into intense exercise. Even engaging in gentle physical activities in, around. and outside the home can be very beneficial.

Practice Relaxation

Stress is an overlooked factor that can disturb your thyroid gland, so it is advisable to set time aside daily for relaxation. Practicing yoga, meditation, or even taking a warm bath can help relieve stress.

If you suspect you might have a thyroid problem, be sure to see your doctor for thyroid testing.

---

55 Bandurska-Stankiewicz, E. (2013). Thyroid hormones – obesity and metabolic syndrome. *Thyroid Research, 6*(Suppl 2), A5. Retrieved from http://www.ncbi.nlm.nih.gov/pmc/articles/PMC3618019/

56 Nomura, M., Tashiro, N., Watanabe, T., Hirata, A., Abe, I., Okabe, T., & Takayanagi, R. (2014). Association of symptoms of gastroesophageal reflux with metabolic syndrome parameters in patients with endocrine disease. *ISRN Gastroenterology, 2104*, 863206. Retrieved from http://www.ncbi.nlm.nih.gov/pmc/articles/PMC3929142/

CHAPTER 27

KEEP A LOG

E ver wonder why you're struggling to lose weight regardless of eating normally? Could you be overeating or eating the wrong foods without knowing it? Keeping a log is a great way to find out how much you actually eat. By logging your daily calories and exercise, you can get a clearer picture of where you might be going wrong and get back on the fast track to weight loss. Just as important, you'll be able to track your successes as well.

A log can be a journal, app, or a sheet of paper where you document what you eat, when you ate it, amount of calories you consume, portions, and calories burned by exercise.

A study coordinated by Kaiser Permanente's Center of Health Research in Portland, Oregon showed that recording daily food and exercise resulted in higher weight losses.[57] Why? Because it allowed dieters to reflect on how much they actually eat every day and to become mindful of eating too much.

Adding exercise to the log makes the technique more effective. By comparing the amount of calories you consume with how much you burn, it is easier to determine if you are gaining weight or losing it.

The more accurate the calories and exercise you record, the better. In addition to tracking calories in meals, you should also count beverages and snacks. Portion sizes are just as important. Underestimating portions is a very common hindrance to weight loss.

To log in physical activity, you first need to know your BMR (basal metabolic rate). This is the number of calories your body burns daily without exercise. A rough estimation of BMR is possible using the Mifflin-St. Jeor equation, which is considered to be the standard when it comes to calculating BMR. It is as follows:

For men: BMR = 4.536 x weight (lbs) + 15.875 x height (in.) – 5 x age (years) + 5

For women: BMR = 4.536 x weight (lbs) + 15.875 x height (in) – 5 x age (years) – 161.

Second, you need to find out how many calories workouts burn. Record both the calories burned and the length of the workout.

If you are prone to emotional eating, jotting down emotions might be very useful. Being aware of the emotions that trigger mindless eating and seeking appropriate help can have a positive effect on your waistline.

You can either created your own log or use online tools or apps that have made logging easier than ever before. There are many health sites that offer free access to weight calculators, food and exercise databases, and calorie count charts for a wide range of foods. You will also be able to get a fairly accurate idea of how many calories you burn by any given exercise or activity.

Ideally, you should log daily. This way, you can track food as you eat. Avoid waiting until the end of the day, if possible, because you might forget important details.

---

57 Kaiser Permanente. (2008). Keeping a food diary doubles diet weight loss, study suggests. *ScienceDaily*. Retrieved from www.sciencedaily.com/releases/2008/07/080708080738.htm

CHAPTER 28

GET A WEIGHT-LOSS BUDDY

A study58 done by the University of Indiana showed that people who choose to share their weight-loss journey with a partner tend to lose more weight than those who don't.

A weight-loss buddy is someone who shares similar goals to yours. It can be a person who wants to lose weight or one who is familiar with the challenges of the journey. This is a person you will be accountable to and vice versa.

Having someone by your side through the ups and downs of losing weight has its benefits. First, it brings accountability, which can help make a challenging diet and fitness routine easier to follow. By committing to certain dietary goals and/or setting times to work out together, both of you are likely to follow through. Accountability is often, in and of itself, the missing link for some people when it comes to sticking to weight-loss goals.

The second benefit of a buddy is emotional support. Stress, disappointment, and frustration are common emotions of weight loss. A partner who has experienced the same obstacles can provide a positive push when needed.

If you are not lucky enough to have friends or family members who want to lose weight, you can always make a new friend. Here are some of the best places to find buddies with similar interests and goals:

The Gym

Your local gym is filled with plenty of potential weight-loss buddies. From personal trainers to first-timers, all you need to do is ask. You might be surprised how many people who, like you, are looking for a buddy.

At Work

This is a great place to find a workout buddy as the workplace is often like a minefield when it comes to healthy eating. Having someone in the same environment who is facing the same challenges can be of great support. You can share healthy snacks and recipes, motivate each other, and support each other when someone brings donuts to a meeting. Great possibilities also exist for going for a walk or exercising together before or after work or at lunch time.

Online

Although it is not as personal as face-to-face interaction, joining an online community can provide great support. There are many websites and online programs where dieters chat, inspire, and exchange recipes with each other. You can also reach out to friends through social media.

---

58 Wallace, J. P. (2005). Twelve month adherence of adults who joined a fitness program with a spouse vs. without a spouse. *Journal of Sports Medicine and Physical Fitness, 33*(3), 206-213. Retrieved from http://www.ncbi.nlm.nih. gov/pubmed?uid=8775648&cmd=showdetailview&indexed=google

CHAPTER 29

MEET WITH AN EXPERT

Whether you are just starting your first diet or you are finding weight loss to be a challenge, meeting with an expert can unlock the secrets to a leaner you. You'll avoid mistakes, get support, and discover how to make the most from your efforts. Nutritionists, personal trainers, and other health experts possess a wealth of knowledge. Here are some benefits of using these professionals:

Personalized Plan

No two bodies are the same. With that said, weight-loss techniques that work for someone else might not be effective for you. Seeing an expert can teach you about what makes your body unique and create a weight-loss strategy that is personalized to your needs.

Work With Your Limitations

An expert can identify and create a plan around your limitations. Whether you are diabetic or physically challenged, a professional can help you work with health conditions, physical limitations, and anything that might hinder weight loss.

Stay Motivated and on Track

It's hard to lose weight alone. This is why you need a support system. A weight-loss expert doubles up as a weight-loss buddy and coach. Experts not only help you overcome challenges but can also cheer you up when you are feeling challenged and help you celebrate your successes as well.

Avoid Common Mistakes

Common mistakes like overtraining or choosing the wrong foods can be easily avoided with advice from a pro. Experts can help you maximize weight-loss results without compromising your health. They also give great tips, supplement recommendations, and effective workouts.

Mix It up

Monotony can make losing weight seem dull and tedious. Having an expert by your side can expose you to a variety of healthy foods, recipes, workouts, and strategies. Eating something new every day or trying new workouts can keep you interested.

Maintain Your Results

Achieving your goal weight is only half of the process. Keeping the pounds off requires some adjustments to your lifestyle.[59] An expert can help you keep the weight off for life and provide new information when you need it.

---

59 Kruger, J., Blanck, H. M., & Gillespie, C. (2006). Dietary and physical activity behaviors among adults successful at weight loss maintenance. *International Journal of Behavioral Nutrition and Physical Activity, 3*(17). Retrieved from http://www.ijbnpa.org/content/3/1/17

CHAPTER 30

GET A FITNESS TRACKER

O f all the weight-loss equipment available today, only a few are as useful and cool as fitness trackers. From counting calories to watching over your heartrate, trackers can provide the "Intel" you need to optimize your efforts.

Fitness trackers have a wide variety of features and can either focus on one task or multitask at the same time, including logging physical activity, calculating calories burned daily, and monitoring your heart beat. Some trackers log the amount of hours you sleep and the number of steps you take (pedometers). Because they resemble wristbands or watches, they are easy to wear, convenient, and inconspicuous.

Additionally, trackers have been shown to have a motivating effect on weight loss, according to a trial published in the *International Journal of Behavioral Nutrition and Physical Activity*.[60] People who regulate their behavior through logging information and reviewing that information, stayed on course and shed more pounds. Monitoring how many calories you burn daily is a great motivator. You can celebrate and reward yourself on days when calorie burn is high. A tracker can also push you to do more on those days you feel less enthusiastic.

Fitness trackers are also useful for people who struggle with logging. Whether you find it tedious or tend to leave out important information, a tracker can record your activity in real time. It takes the stress out of logging by simplifying the task. By using one, you'll gain a clearer perspective on your weight-loss strategies, instant feedback, and the information you need to achieve better results.

There are a variety of fitness trackers available at various price points, some of which give you a trial period to see if you like using it. So give it a go. Who knows? Your fitness tracker might just be your new fitness buddy!

---

60   Gokee-LaRose, J., Gorin, A. A., & Wing, R. R. (2009). Behavioral self-regulation for weight loss in young adults: A randomized controlled trial. *International Journal of Behavioral Nutrition and Physical Activity 6*(10). Retrieved from http://www.ijbnpa.org/content/6/1/10

CHAPTER 31

EAT 4-6 SMALLER MEALS A DAY

Many people grew up on three solid square meals a day, and maybe a snack or two in between. That's perfectly okay. But if you are trying to lose weight and stay in shape, you might need to consider splitting your meals into 4-6 portions with breakfast as the biggest meal. Why?

An interesting study published by the International Congress of Nutrition revealed that eating more frequently can help you slim down. Experts noticed that participants who had a fourth meal had healthier BMIs than those who ate three meals a day.[61]

In addition to improving your energy, curbing hunger, and boosting metabolism, eating more frequently has been shown to regulate insulin. Insulin is important to weight loss because it controls the amount of sugar in the body. When insulin response is healthy, sugar is metabolized instead of being stored as fat.

In addition having 4-6 meals a day it is very helpful to eat a bigger breakfast as well. Eating more calories at breakfast has been shown to result in greater weight loss and inches lost around the waist.62 It also normalizes blood sugar and insulin for stable energy and reduces the fats that can cause heart disease. (See the chapter "Eat a Big Breakfasts" for more on this subject.)

To make the most of this slimming technique, determine how many calories you need in order to lose weight. Divide those calories into 5-6 meals, making sure breakfast has a higher calorie count.

---

61 Louis-Sylvestre, J., Llunch, A., Neant, F., & Blundell, J. E. (2003). Highlighting the positive impact of increasing feeding frequency on metabolism and weight management. *Forum Nutrition, 56*, 126-128. Retrieved from http://www.ncbi.nlm.nih.gov/pubmed/15806828?ordinalpos=1&itool=EntrezSystem2.PEntrez.Pubmed.Pubmed_ResultsPanel.Pubmed_SingleItemSupl.Pubmed_Discovery_RA&linkpos=5&log$=relatedreviews&logdbfrom=pubmed

62 Jakubowicz, D., Barnea, M., Wainstein, J., & Froy, O. (2013). High caloric intake at breakfast vs. dinner differentially influences weight loss of overweight and obese women. *Obesity, 21*(12), 2504-2512. Retrieved from http://www.ncbi.nlm.nih.gov/pubmed/23512957

CHAPTER 32

SNEAK A LITTLE ACTIVITY IN YOUR LIFE

E very activity burns a certain amount of calories, some more than others. Even simple actions like walking, dancing, and gentle stretching can give your metabolism a quick boost. Whether you're at home or at work, there are many ways to sneak activity into your schedule, which will give a boost to your weight-loss efforts.

At Home

There are many tasks you can do around the house to increase your daily calorie burn. Cleaning, washing your car, and gardening can burn hundreds of calories per hour. You can also get a nice mini workout by cleaning out your closet, sweeping the driveway, taking the dog for a nice walk, or raking leaves in the backyard.

Another way to sneak in some physical activity is by stretching and standing while watching TV. A study in the *Journal of Pediatric Psychology* found that watching television might increase the risk of weight gain.[63] Therefore, make an effort to get off the couch once in a while and find something physical to do, and I don't mean walking to the kitchen to get another snack. Try standing and sitting repeatedly, several times during the commercial breaks.

At Work

There are plenty of opportunities to squeeze in a little activity on your way to and from work as well as at the office. If you drive or take the bus to work, try riding a bike. You can also get off at the stop before your usual one and take a walk.

When you get to the office, ditch the elevator and opt for stairs instead. During your lunch break, walk to the store or run errands on foot. With little effort, you can get your heart pumping and burn a few calories. It will be good for your energy too!

In Your Spare Time

You can burn calories and fat while having a good time by finding a hobby or activity you enjoy. Here are some ideas to get you started: take dance lessons, join a ping pong club, go swimming, meet a neighbor for a walk, go for a bike ride, take in a museum, etc. The more enjoyable the activity, the more you are likely to do it.

Being active doesn't always have to involve intense exercise. Engaging in simple physical activities every day can have huge benefits for your figure, health, and well-being.

---

63   *Danner, F. W. (2008). A national longitudinal study of the association between hours of TV viewing and the trajectory of BMI growth among US children. Journal of Pediatric Psychology, 33, 1100-1107. Retrieved from* http://www.ncbi.nlm.nih.gov/pubmed/18390579

CHAPTER 33

ENJOY MORE SOUP

Slurping soup is not just good for when you are feeling under the weather; it can help you lose weight too. Low in calories and full of rich flavor, soup might just be the weight-loss ally you've been looking for.

Soup has a high water percentage and foods that contain a lot of water are very filling as well as a low calorie count. In fact, a study published in the journal *Appetite* revealed that liquids can be more satisfying than solid food.[64]

Another valuable benefit of soup is that it can help you eat less throughout the day. The same study mentioned above shows that people who eat soup as a main meal tend to consume fewer calories after that. For instance, if you decide on soup for lunch, it is likely you will choose a smaller dinner. Of course, you can have a bowl of soup before a meal as a way of curbing your appetite.

In addition to facilitating weight loss, soup can give you a nutritional boost. Depending on what you add to it, your broth can be a good source of important vitamins and minerals.

Unfortunately not every soup is good for weight loss. There is a big calorie and nutritional difference between vegetable broth and a creamy chowder, for example. The best soups are those that are broth-based and contain plenty of fresh vegetables, legumes, and beans.

You should also be careful when using bouillon cubes. Although they add flavor, they are also very high in sodium. Too much sodium in your system can cause high blood pressure.

---

64   Flood, J. E., & Rolls, B. J. (2007). Soup preloads in a variety of forms reduce energy intake. *Appetite 49*(3), 626-634. Retrieved from http://www.ncbi.nlm. nih.gov/pmc/articles/PMC2128765/

CHAPTER 34

SET REALISTIC GOALS

M aking the decision to lose weight is great. However, in order to achieve weight loss and stay motivated, it is important to set realistic goals.[65] Instead of trying to shed as many pounds as possible, it is advisable to take a step back and think about what is possible and what is not.

A weight-loss goal is realistic if it is achievable without comprising your health. More often than not, people fall into the trap of wanting to lose as much weight as possible quickly. Keep in mind that if you lose more than a couple of pounds each week, you risk losing muscle that you want to keep because it helps burn calories. It is also hard to gain the muscle back once you lose it, while it is much easier to gain fat. Studies also show that those who lose weight slowly over time are most likely to keep the weight off.

It's also common for people to pull out their college pictures and use them as motivation to lose weight. However, "trying to get your body back" can be unachievable and even dangerous to your health. Instead of stepping back in time, focus on the present. Lose weight to look good with the body you have now.

Another element to factor into your goal-setting process is sustainability. Is your ideal weight sustainable? Can you follow the same diet and exercise routine you used to get to that weight for life? When deciding on your goal weight, make sure you are prepared to maintain it.

WHAT ARE REALISTIC WEIGHT-LOSS GOALS?

Body Mass Index (BMI)

A method that can help you set achievable goals is the Body Mass Index. BMI consists of four categories: healthy, underweight, overweight, and obese. If you fall within the last two categories, focus on losing enough weight to be in the healthy range. Online calculators are available to help you determine your current BMI.

Frame, Age, and Gender

When setting goals, you should also consider your frame, age, and gender. These factors play a critical role in how much weight you can actually lose. If you have a large frame, for instance, it is not realistic to expect to weigh as much as a person with a smaller frame.

Age and gender also influence metabolism. Generally, the older you get, the more challenging losing weight is. You might not lose weight in your 40s as fast as you did in your 20s. When it comes to gender, female bodies tend to hold onto fat more than their male counterparts.

---

65 Wamsteker, E. W., Geenen, R., Zelissen, P. M., Van Furth, E. F., & Lestra, J. (2009). Unrealistic weight-loss goals among obese patients are associated with age and causal attributions. *Journal of the American Dietetic Association 109*(11), 1903-1908. Retrieved from http://www.ncbi.nlm.nih.gov/pubmed/19857632

CHAPTER 35

OUT OF SIGHT – OUT OF MOUTH!

Are you familiar with the old saying "out of sight, out of mind"? The same holds true for food. What you see, you want more of; what you don't see, you think less about. Since most of losing weight is about controlling your diet, it might be wise to start putting away unhealthy foods and setting your sights on healthier options.

Research studies by Ohio State University show a link between where people place food in their homes and their food choices. Those who had unhealthy foods visibly placed and readily accessible weighed more and were at greater risk of becoming obese.[66]

With that said, in order to lose weight successfully, you need to place fattening foods where you see them less often. You also need to create "obstacles" between you and the foods. Examples of creating obstacles include placing them on the highest shelf in the kitchen, or sealing and placing them behind other foods.

The more challenging it is to reach the foods, the better you will be able to control your cravings. You might also consider not even bringing them into your home; if they are not there, you won't be tempted to eat them.

Generally, foods that should be out of sight include high-carb snacks and those high in sugars. This can be anything from a chocolate bar to potato chips. You can take it a step further and include all processed, high-calorie foods you find hard to resist.

Making unhealthy foods less visible is a particularly useful technique to use if members of your household are not on a diet. Whether your spouse has a goody cabinet or your kids have the habit of leaving food around the house, this method can help you stick to your weight-loss plan.

Alternatively, you can encourage your partner, friends, and family to join in your quest to live healthier. At the very least, you can ask them for their support as you are working to achieve your weight-loss goals.

Next time you go grocery shopping, make a list of healthy foods and leave treats on the store shelf where they belong. Remember, not buying unhealthy foods in the first place is the most effective way to keep them out of sight and out of mouth.

---

66   Emery, C. F., Olson, K. L., Lee, V. S., Habash, D. L., Nasar, J. L., & Bodine, A. (2015). **Home environment and psychosocial predictors of obesity status among community-residing men and women.** *International Journal of Obesity, 28.*

CHAPTER 36

DO A LITTLE PLANNING

Have you noticed that almost every diet comes with a meal plan, a detailed menu of what you will eat for breakfast, lunch, and supper. Why? Because planning meals in advance helps you stay on track, stay within calorie limit, and shed more pounds.[67] This strategy has been proven to maximize weight loss. Here are the reasons why:

Anticipate Your Calories

One of the benefits of meal planning is being able to produce a menu that fits your caloric intake. For instance, if you are on a 1,500-calorie diet, planning helps you distribute these calories between main meals, snacks, and drinks. When you eat as you go, you're more likely to exceed your limit than when you plan ahead.

Control Portions Better

Portion control goes hand in hand with calorie count. If you underestimate portions, you will inevitably underestimate the amount of calories you eat as well. Planning meals in advance gives you time to measure portions better than eating on the run.

Eliminate Guesswork

Another advantage of planning ahead is not having to worry about what you're going to eat all day. This is especially beneficial if you're not accustomed to cooking healthy, calorie-controlled meals.

Expose Mindless Eating

Without a meal plan, you run the risk of piling on calories through mindless eating. Mindless eating can be the bagel you grab on the way to work, that occasional energy drink, and all the other calories that are adding to your intake you're not aware of.

Make Better Food Choices

When you have a tight calorie budget to work with, you are more likely to make better food choices. In the process of trying to keep meals as low-calorie as possible, choosing healthy foods like lean proteins and fruits and vegetables is inevitable.

Make Better Use of Your Time

By planning meals in advance, you can also plan for the ingredients you need for several meals. Make an effort to prepare enough food so that you can have it for several meals during the week. Freeze some, and you have healthy and delicious food ready when you need it. This is also good time management!

MEAL PLANNING TIPS

The easiest way to start is by browsing for free meal plans online. There are hundreds, if not thousands, of meal plans out there. Choose one according to your recommended calorie intake. For more flexibility, you can purchase cookbooks with healthy recipes. Look for books with calorie counts of each meal to create your meal plan.

Another option is to create your own recipes. For beginners, this might be challenging at first but gets easier over time. You can check the calorie count of ingredients used with an online food database for accuracy.

Planning meals in advance also means planning your portions too. If you haven't yet got the hang of eyeballing portions, you can use other techniques like using smaller plates or comparing food portions to certain objects (tennis ball, deck of cards, etc.).

---

67 Center for Disease Control and Prevention. (2011). Planning
    Meals. Retrieved from http://www.cdc.gov/healthyweight/healthy_
    eating/meals.html

CHAPTER 37

STAY MOTIVATED

The idea of losing weight is exciting. The thought of looking and feeling great is enough to get you off the couch. But what happens when the enthusiasm fizzles out? It might be an oversimplification to say you need to stay motivated, but that is exactly what needs to happen. A little thought and planning will help you stay focused and on track toward your weight-loss goals. Here are some ways you can overcome common obstacles and stay motivated:

Know the Benefits

There are so many other advantages to losing weight than just looking great. If improving your appearance is not enough to keep you going, focus on what shedding pounds will do for your health, and self-esteem. From gaining confidence to reducing the risk of chronic conditions, list all the benefits waiting for you at the finish line. Write these down and post them in conspicuous places where you will see them daily.

Find Like-Minded People

One of the best ways to stay motivated is to find a weight-loss buddy. Whether it's a pal from work, a friend from the gym, or your spouse, having someone with similar goals by your side can renew your enthusiasm. If finding a buddy proves too challenging, you can find support online or sign up for a weight-loss challenge.

Set Achievable Goals

Many people make the error of setting unrealistic weight-loss goals and becoming discouraged when they don't achieve them. Instead of trying to lose massive amounts of weight in a short time, focus on losing 1-2 pounds per week. (See the chapter on "Setting Realistic Goals")

Reward Yourself for Achieving Milestones

A good way to stay excited is to create weight-loss milestones and reward yourself for achieving them. Milestones can be weekly, biweekly, or monthly. Work out how much weight you can lose in a period of time. When you do, treat yourself to a spa, weekend vacation, or anything else you enjoy, except unhealthy food. (See Chapter 43, Reward Yourself.)

Go by Inches and Not Numbers

Contrary to popular belief, the scale is not always a good indicator of your progress. In fact, as you gain muscle mass, you might weigh more.[68] This is why it is advisable to go by measurements instead of numbers. Measure your waist, hips, and arms to get more accurate results.

Do What You Like

It is easier to stick to a diet or follow a fitness routine if you enjoy it. Instead of serving bland meals or repeating workouts, jazz up your weight-loss plan with new recipes and try different workouts. When you find what you love, staying motivated won't be a problem.

Model Success

Talk to others who have successfully lost weight. Ask them how they did it? What secrets can they offer? What did they do when they became challenged—how did they overcome it? What were their key success strategies? It has been said, "success leaves clues." It can also be inspiring just to speak with someone who has achieved similar goals to yours.

Go Easy on Yourself

One of the biggest obstacles you can face on your weight-loss journey is—you. Being critical of yourself when you don't achieve your goals can dampen your mood fast. Focus on small achievements, the first being that you made the decision to lose weight and take control of your health.

---

68   Titchenal, A., & Dobbs, J. (2002, January 9). Exercise program can result in quick weight gain. *Honolulu Star-Bulletin*. Retrieved from http://www.nutritionatc.hawaii.edu/HO/2002/135.htm

CHAPTER 38

GO SHOPPING WITH A LIST

When you're in the process of losing weight, a visit to the supermarket can either make or break your success. Grocery stores are filled with foods that can easily lead you astray. Taking a shopping list can help you stay focused on your weight-loss path and resist the many temptations in the aisles.

A shopping list plays a huge role in the food choices you make at the store, and by following one, you can dramatically increase your chances for weight-loss success. Here are some of the ways a list can boost your weight-loss efforts:

Prevents Impulse Purchases

Supermarkets profit on impulse purchases, and you are likely to make them if you are not shopping for something specific. Arming yourself with a shopping list keeps you focused on what you need. It helps you avoid distractions and reduces the impulse to grab unhealthy goodies on your way to the check-out lane.[69]

Prevents Bad Food Choices

When you go to the store without a plan, you double the likelihood of making poor food choices. Although most people know to avoid sugar-loaded and high-carb foods like chips and ice cream, other food options might appear healthy when they actually are not. Planning your list will help you avoid these items.

Prevents Buying More Than You Need

Many people get discouraged about following a healthy diet because it seems expensive. It doesn't have to be. Instead of piling your cart with anything and everything healthy, compiling a food list for the week will give you great control over how much to buy.

WHAT SHOULD BE ON THE SHOPPING LIST?

A great way to narrow down your shopping list is to plan meals for multiple days. There are many websites that offer sample menus for weight loss as well as healthy recipe. Once you have your menu, go shopping only for those ingredients.

If you prefer crafting your own meals, the best options to include in your list are fresh fruits, vegetables, legumes, whole grains, dairy, healthy fats like olive oil or coconut oil, chicken, turkey, fish and lean meats (or vegetarian proteins). Shop for organic foods if possible and avoid processed foods that carry empty calories. Almost everything in a package is processed—so read labels carefully!

69 Fielding-Singh, P., Almy, J., & Wootan, M. (2014). Sugar overload: Retail checkout promotes obesity. Center for Science in the Public Interest. Retrieved from http://cspinet.org/sugaroverload.pdf

CHAPTER 39

MAKE THE SMOOTHIE SWITCH

Nutritious, delicious, and easy to whip up, smoothies are a welcome addition to any diet. Replacing one meal or snack a day with a smoothie is a habit that can cut down your calories, help you lose extra pounds, and keep you lean for years.[70]

You make smoothies with unprocessed natural ingredients that you choose, so they make excellent low-calorie meals. In addition, smoothies are dense in nutrients; vitamins and minerals are essential to metabolic function. If you add plenty of protein and fiber, you can also effectively control your appetite.

Like any balanced meal, weight-loss smoothies should include healthy amounts of protein, fiber, and good fats. It is also wise to include as many essential vitamins and minerals as possible. Organic foods like fruit, vegetables, nuts, seeds, and dairy are ideal ingredients because they contain the nutrients needed to boost weight loss.

If you would like to substitute your normal breakfast with a smoothie, use ingredients that are high in protein and fiber. Filling up on protein early can control your appetite for hours and help you eat fewer calories throughout the day.

You can make a simple breakfast smoothie by blending:

- **2 cups of low-fat milk or milk substitute like almond or rice milk**
- **½ cup plain Greek yogurt**
- **½ cup of blueberries or mixed berries**
- **A handful of almonds**
- **A handful of ice cubes**

You can swap berries for any other fruit like a banana or apple. You can also switch almonds for any other type of nuts.

Vegetable smoothies also make great meal replacements, are filling, contain less sugar, and are low in calories. If you've never made a green smoothie before, try this easy recipe.

Blend:

- **1 cup of spinach or kale**
- **1 cup apple juice**
- **1 cup ice**
- **½ banana**

- 1/2 tablespoon crunchy peanut butter
- ½ tablespoon flaxseeds

If you find the taste of leafy greens overwhelming, here is another green recipe you might find more appetizing:

- 1 avocado (medium)
- ½ cup spinach leaves (You won't even know they are there!)
- 1 banana
- 1 ½ cups soy or almond milk
- ½ cup mango slices or papaya
- ½ teaspoon honey or vanilla extract

Here is a smoothie recipe for chocolate lovers:

- 1 cup light coconut milk
- 1 teaspoon honey
- ¼ cup water (or more according to desired consistency)
- 2 tablespoons chocolate-flavored protein powder

The recipes above are ideas just to get you started. There are literally hundreds of ingredient combinations to try. When in doubt, remember to always include:

- ☐ A cup of liquid
- ☐ A cup of ice
- ☐ A fruit
- ☐ A portion of nuts or seeds

☐ A cup of leafy vegetable (optional)

---

70 Heymsfield, S. B., van Mierlo, C. A. J., van der Knaap, H. C. M., Heo, M., &
    Frier, H. I. (2003). Weight management using a meal replacement strategy:
    Meta and pooling analysis from six studies. *International Journal of Obesity,*
    27, 537-549. Retrieved from http://www.nature.com/ijo/journal/v27/n5/
    full/0802258a.html

CHAPTER 40

HAVE A LITTLE PROTEIN WITH EVERY MEAL OR SNACK

O nce upon a time, protein was considered a nutrient only athletes needed. As scientific research unraveled, it became clear how important protein is to weight loss and maintaining a healthy body.[71] Having a little protein with your meals and snacks can help you feel satiated and energized all day long. Adequate protein diets have been shown to be effective at speeding up the weight-loss process. Here are some of the ways protein affects body and weight-loss efforts:

Fill Up on Less

Foods high in protein are not only satiating, they can also decrease your appetite. This is because they allow leptin to send your brain signals faster. Leptin is the hormone that tells your brain whether you are full and to stop eating or you're not full and you should eat more.

As your leptin response improves, you will be able to feel satisfied with less food. In other words, it helps you manage your calories naturally.[72]

Keeps Your Liver Busy

The liver performs many tasks and one of them is breaking down fats, carbs, and protein. If the liver is not working at its best, it can cause fat to build up around your midsection. Feeding this vital organ with a high-protein diet keeps it busy and consequently raises your metabolism.

Take Care of Muscle

Muscle burns energy, and the higher your muscle mass, the faster your metabolism. Muscle, however, is not self-sustaining. It requires plenty of protein from your diet to stay in optimal condition. If your diet is low in protein, muscle is likely to erode over time and, with it, your ability to burn calories effectively.

HOW MUCH PROTEIN DO YOU NEED?

The U.S. Department of Agriculture recommends that all men and women over the age of 19 get at least 0.37 grams per pound. For example, a woman who is 130 pounds should get at least 48 grams of protein, a 200 pound man should get 74 grams of protein. Keep in mind that these are minimums, and if you exercise regularly or are an athlete, you may require up to twice these amounts. What is most important for weight loss is making sure that you are having some protein with every meal and every snack. This will help keep the hunger gremlins away!

Good protein snacks include a handful of almonds, a piece of cheese, a couple slices of turkey, peanut butter, yogurt (watch the sugar though), or a protein smoothie. And, of course, at meal times, you will want to include high-quality protein sources such as fish, chicken, turkey, lamb, and lean cuts of pork and beef.

A word of caution, although adding protein is a good idea, too much of a good thing can be bad for your health. Excessive consumption of protein has been linked to kidney stones, gout, yeast and bacterial infections, weight gain, and cancer. So it is best to stick to the recommended intake.

---

71 Paddon-Jones, D., Westman, E., Mattes, R. D., Wolfe, R. R., Astrup, A., & Westerterp-Plantenga, M. (2008). Protein, weight management and satiety. *American Journal of Clinical Nutrition 87*(5), 1558S-1561S. Retrieved from http://www.ncbi.nlm.nih.gov/pubmed/18469287

72 Weigle, D. S., Breen, P. A., Matthys, C. C., Callahan, H. S., Meeuws, K. E., Burden, V. R., & Purnell, J. Q. (2005). A high-protein diet induces sustained reductions in appetite, ad libitum caloric intake, and body weight despite compensatory changes in diurnal plasma leptin and ghrelin concentrations. *American Journal of Clinical Nutrition 82*(1), 41-48. Retrieved from http://www.ncbi.nlm.nih.gov/pubmed/16002798

CHAPTER 41

THE 12-HOUR FAST

In the past few years, weight loss diets that involve controlled fasting have caught the attention of dieters. But can you really lose weight by fasting for just 12 hours every day?

At the most basic level, "intermittent fasting" is intentionally going without food for a specific period of time. This period can range anywhere between a few days and a few hours.

Being on a 12-hour fast diet means you won't be eating for 12 hours. This could be 7 p.m. to 7 a.m., for example, or whatever time suits your schedule. During the fast, you are only allowed foods with little or no calories, like water. This eating pattern is then repeated daily to accelerate weight loss.

The science behind this technique is relatively simple. One of the causes of weight gain is eating more sugars than you burn. And it takes 8-12 hours for the body to fully use sugars as energy. By eating at certain intervals, you starve your body of sugars, and it will have no other option but to start burning fat as an energy source.

To successfully lose weight by fasting, you need to make sure there is a 12-hour window between meals. The second guideline to weight-loss fasting is to pay attention to what you eat. During the non-fasting periods, it is best to choose foods high in nutrients. Supplying your body with enough vitamins, minerals, fiber, and protein will improve energy levels and ensure you're burning maximum calories.

The third guideline is optional but recommended. Adding exercise to intermittent fasting can give you greater results. However, do not overdo it. Engage in less strenuous activity like household chores, taking walks, and standing instead of sitting to burn extra calories on the side.

There is scientific evidence that intermittent fasting is good for your health.[73] When done right, you can lose those stubborn pounds and feel energized in the process. Remember to consult your doctor first if you have any existing health conditions.

---

73   Murray, U. T. (2011, March 04). Study finds routine periodic fasting is good for your health, and your heart. *Eureka Alert*. Retrieved from http://www.eurekalert.org/pub_releases/2011-04/imc-sfr033111.php

CHAPTER 42

TRY YOGA

Recent scientific research has shown that middle-aged people who practice yoga regularly gain less weight during their middle years than those who don't. According to a multi-year research study by the Fred Hutchinson Cancer Research Center, those practicing yoga for 10 years between ages 45 and 55 lost five pounds on average, while those who did not gained 14 pounds.[74]

Here are some ways that yoga can help you lose weight:

Tones the Glandular System:

It is believed that yoga helps to tone the glandular system, including the thyroid and parathyroid, which are the master glands of metabolism. Your thyroid and parathyroid are located in your throat area and are affected by various postures.

Improves Digestion

Most postures and yogic breathing techniques (pranayama) also affect the digestive tract by toning the organs of the stomach, thereby improving nutritional absorption of food as well as aiding in elimination.

Burns Calories

Whether it is gentle yoga or a more vigorous practice, movement burns calories. And as anyone who has taken Ashtanga Yoga or a flow style yoga class can tell you—yoga can be quite aerobic. Yoga also helps to build muscle, which helps to burn calories. Poses such plank, downward facing dog, handstand, and balancing poses are all good examples of strength-building postures. The more you work on your strength, the more muscle you will build. The more muscle you have, the more your body will burn calories—even when resting!

Increase Body Awareness

Many overweight people are disconnected from their body. Slowly and gradually, yoga helps you tune in and connect with your body so that you're better able to understand its cues. You're better able to identify when you're hungry and when you're feeling something else. What's more, yoga helps you feel better in your body: improving circulation, enhancing flexibility, and clearing your mind.

Balances Emotions and Reduces Stress

There are numerous emotional reasons why people overeat. Some of the more common ones include trying to fill a void, using food to numb oneself, mediating stress or anxiety levels, or having a hard time being present. Of course, this just a partial list of emotional reasons why people overeat. Yoga helps to balance emotions, which helps you to feel good about yourself. And when you feel good about yourself, you are less likely to overeat for emotional reasons. The practice of yoga brings us deep inside to a place where we can know that everything is okay—to a place of peace and connection to something larger. Equally important, yoga teaches you to accept yourself right where you are at this place in time—without judgment.

---

74 Kristal, A. R., Littman, A. J., Benitez, D., & White, E. (2005). Yoga practice is associated with attenuated weight gain in healthy middle-aged men and women. *Alternative Therapies in Health and Medicine 11*(4), 28-33. Retrieved from http://www.ncbi.nlm.nih.gov/pubmed/16053119

CHAPTER 43

REWARD YOURSELF

Celebrating small successes by rewarding yourself is a great way to spike your motivation and drive to achieve weight-loss goals.[75] By identifying rewards, not only will you have something fun to look forward to, but you will be recognizing and acknowledging your success.

There are plenty of ways to give yourself a pat on the back for losing weight. Here are just some ideas you can add to your list for achieving your next milestone. Consider big rewards for long-term goals and smaller rewards for short-term goals (weekly or biweekly). Both are important!

Here are some ideas to get your started:

Pamper Your Body

Spoil your body with a trip to the spa, or schedule a massage.

Buy Something for Your New Look

Your body is changing, why not your look? Reward yourself with a new pair of jeans, buy new gym clothes, or change your hair color. Working on a new look can get you excited about your progress and what's to come.

Capture and Share Your Progress

Seeing a before and after picture of yourself can rekindle your commitment to the process. Get a family member or friend to take full-length photos. Take it a step further and share the pictures with your personal and social network.

Gain Helpful Skills and Get New Gadgets

Why not invest in skills and gadgets to make weight loss more fun? Try out new recipes, take a cooking class, get a heart-rate monitor, or buy exercise equipment. There are countless gadgets and classes that are fun, useful, and cost-effective.

Other good ideas for rewards include theater tickets, weekend getaways, a day off from work, a new haircut, a fresh bouquet of flowers, a new pair of shoes, etc.

Be careful in creating rewards not to use unhealthy food as a reward because this can harm your efforts in the long term. Valuing fattening or unhealthy foods only makes them more attractive. It also promotes a negative attitude toward healthy living and makes it difficult to let them go.

75 National Heart, Lung, and Blood Institute. (n.d.). Guide to behavior change. Retrieved from https://www.nhlbi.nih.gov/health/educational/lose_wt/behavior.htm

CHAPTER 44

SHOP AT FARMERS MARKETS

Next time you go grocery shopping, why not take a detour through the farmers market? Filled with fresh, healthy, and affordable foods, farmers markets are a paradise for anyone trying to lose weight by improving food choices.[76] You can find almost every kind of food at markets. While some sell mainly fruits and vegetables, others sell a blend of crops, meats, and even seafood, grains, nuts, and seeds. Instead of sending it to grocery stores, farmers display their wares in public so people can purchase fresher food directly at lower prices; food comes straight from the farm to your table. Here are some of the many benefits of shopping at a farmers market:

Fresh Foods

Farmers markets are all about fresh foods, many of them organically grown. From crispy greens to seasonal fruits to unprocessed meats, you can find a wide variety fresh, nutritious foods. And because the food is fresher, it maintains more of its nutrition and great taste.

Natural Low-Calorie Options

Calories are one less thing to worry about when you visit a farmers market. Fresh produce is naturally low in calories and much more satiating than their processed counterparts. With no hidden carbs, sugars, or unhealthy fats, fresh food tastes great and is good for you too!

Affordable Healthy Living

One of the biggest challenges of living healthy is the cost of buying organic. Because the foods at farmers markets do not need to be transported or packaged before arriving on your dinner table, they are usually at a better price than in the grocery stores.

Menu Inspiration

The market is a great place to find inspiration for new healthy recipes. In addition to commonly enjoyed foods, there are also many seasonal and exotic options to try. Experimenting with new foods can keep you excited about cooking healthy and help you stay on the weight-loss track.

Mingle with Like-Minded People

Food is not the only thing you'll find at farmers markets. It is also a great place to make friends and get to know the farmers—the people who have grown your food!

---

76 Jillcott Pitts, S. B., Wu, Q., Demarest, C. L., Dixona, C. E., Dortchea, C. J. M., Bullock, S. L.... Ammermana, A. S. (2015). Farmers market shopping and dietary behaviors among supplemental nutrition assistance program participants. *Public Health Nutrition, 1*(6), 1-8. Retrieved from http://journals.cambridge.org/action/displayAbstract?fromPage=online&aid=9667845&fileId=S1368980015001111

CHAPTER 45

ACUPUNCTURE: GET THE POINT

A cupuncture is an ancient Chinese medical practice that has been used to cure all kinds of ailments. It is primarily performed by inserting needles into different parts of the body that affect and direct healing energy.

According to a clinical trial in the *International Journal of Obesity,* patients who underwent acupuncture sessions saw better and faster weight-loss results.[77]

By inserting a few needles in the auricular or ear area, the practice was shown to have a positive effect on weight loss.[78] Acupuncture focused on the ear decreased appetite, which means it can help you eat less, particularly helpful if you struggle with controlling your hunger. It is believed that the acupuncture treatment affects the rate of metabolism, your body's ability to burn fuel.

Acupuncture can also help with weight loss by improving your mood and reducing stress, which is directly related to emotional eating.

---

77 Cho, S. H., Lee, J. S., Thabane, L., & Lee, J. (2009). Acupuncture for obesity: A systematic review and meta-analysis. *International Journal of Obesity 33*(2), 183-196. Retrieved from http://www.ncbi.nlm.nih.gov/pubmed/19139756#

78 Ito, H., Yamada, O., Kira, Y., Tanaka, T., & Matsuoka, R. (2015). The effects of auricular acupuncture on weight reduction and feeding related cytokines: A pilot study. *BMJ Open Gastroenterology 2*: e000013. Retrieved from http://bmjopengastro.bmj.com/doi/full/10.1136/bmjgast-2014-000013

CHAPTER 46

CHANGE ONE THING PER WEEK

Making changes to your lifestyle at a steady pace has been shown to be more effective than rapid weight-loss efforts in the long run.[79] In other words, people who lose weight by making changes all at once tend to gain back the pounds eventually. On the other hand, those who make gradual change have a higher success rate with lifelong weight management.

There are many habits and small changes you can incorporate into your lifestyle to achieve lasting weight loss and good health. Here are some easy ways to get started.

Shave Off Calories

You can make living on fewer calories tolerable by shaving 100 calories off your daily count each week until you reach your calorie or weight-loss goal. This way, your body will adjust and you will keep hunger under control.

A common error that people make in an effort to lose weight quickly is to eat as few calories as possible. Some go to the extent of trying to survive on a few bites of food each day. Unfortunately, starving yourself will only stir up hunger and lead to binge eating.

Make Food Substitutes

A great small change to make every week is to trade in a fattening food for a healthier option. You can substitute foods with little nutrition for satiating foods with plenty of vitamins, minerals, protein, and fiber. For example, trade low-fat yogurt for sour cream,

Pick a Veggie

As nutritious and low-calorie as they are, many people still struggle with eating enough vegetables every day. You can make it easier by adding one more vegetable to your menu per day per week until you are eating 7-9 servings of vegetables per day.

Just Add Water

Drinking more water is a lifestyle change that benefits both your figure and health in general. If you are not used to drinking 8-12 glasses of water every day, start by adding at least one glass of water per day per week until you reach 8 glasses per day. (See the chapter Stay Hydrated for more information.)

Adopt Other Fat-Burning Habits

Habits like eating a big breakfast, getting at least 7 hours of uninterrupted sleep, increasing your fiber intake, and reducing stress can make a big difference to your weight. Not only do they trim your figure but they also improve your overall well-being.

---

79 Hill, J. O. (2009). Can a small-changes approach help address the obesity epidemic? A report of the Joint Task Force of the American Society for Nutrition, Institute of Food Technologists, and International Food Information Council. *American Society of Nutrition.* Retrieved from http://ajcn.nutrition.org/content/89/2/477.full.pdf+html

CHAPTER 47

EAT AT HOME MORE OFTEN

E ating out is common for many of us, especially when we're busy and have little or no time to cook. Unfortunately though, this convenience might be packing on the pounds or making it hard to reach your weight-loss goals. The thought of having your favorite meal ready in minutes without ever stepping into the kitchen is very appetizing. However, eating out has its consequences. Instead of blowing your calorie budget as well as your financial budget dining at restaurants, it might be wiser to stay in and eat at home. Here's why:

More Calories

Did you know that people tend to eat more at restaurants than at home? Studies show that the average person consumes more calories eating out than they do when staying in, especially if they eat at buffets.[80]

Poor Quality Calories

In addition to eating more calories, the quality of those calories is also a big question. This is because many restaurant meals have a high amount of sugar and fat. These meals are often high in sodium as well.

Super-Sized Portions

Portions are another problem with eating out. Meal portions have increased significantly over the years.[81] Larger portions mean more calories.

Alcohol

Restaurants are social settings. Having a few drinks with a meal is not uncommon. Unfortunately, alcohol drinks contain plenty of empty calories. Alcohol is also known to slow down the metabolism, which can sabotage your efforts to lose weight.

Desserts

Almost every restaurant offers desserts and they are not shy about it either. Some places actually roll the dessert cart up to your table or put a dessert menu on the table or in your hands! It can be hard to resist these temptations when placed right in front of you.

HOW WILL YOU LOSE WEIGHT BY EATING AT HOME?

Eating at home can help you lose more weight because you are in control of the ingredients you use, the amount of calories in your meals, and the quality of those calories. Preparing your own healthy meals at home makes it easier to keep track of caloric intake. It also helps you avoid hidden oils and sugars that are so commonly used in restaurants.

Enjoying meals at home also gives you advantage over portions. You can effectively control portions by weighing food, using smaller plate sizes, and reading food labels.

---

80 McCrory, M. A., Fuss, P. J., Hays, N. P., Vinken, A. G., Greenberg, A. S., & Roberts, S. B. (1999). Overeating in America: Association between restaurant food consumption and body fatness in healthy adult men and women. *Obesity Research* 7(6), 564-571. Retrieved from http://onlinelibrary.wiley.com/doi/10.1002/j.1550-8528.1999.tb00715.x/abstract

81 Young, L. R., & Nestle, M. (2002). The contribution of expanding portion sizes to the US obesity epidemic. *American Journal of Public Health* 92(2), 246-249. Retrieved from http://www.ncbi.nlm.nih.gov/pmc/articles/PMC1447051/

CHAPTER 48

EAT SLOWLY

Many people don't realize how fast they actually eat and how much it influences their appetite. It takes 20 minutes for your brain to realize you're full.[82] Unfortunately, by then, you may have finished your meal and are probably going for seconds. By taking the time to let your brain register the signals from your stomach, you can feel full on fewer calories and lose more weight.

There is no recommended pace for chewing your food, but there are strategies to help you slow down:

Avoid Eating On-The-Go

If you are one of those people who has a hectic schedule, then eating on the go seems normal. Next time you grab a meal, while rushing out the door, don't eat it right away. Wait until you're in a setting that allows you to eat for at least 20 minutes.

Schedule Eating Times

Another way to slow down is to have specific mealtimes. Whether you're at home or work, setting time aside to eat properly can yield weight-loss benefits in the long term.

Don't Wait for Hunger to Build Up

If scheduling mealtimes is too rigid for your routine, the alternative is to start eating (slowly) when hunger strikes. Postponing a meal only builds up hunger pangs, which will cause you to wolf down food later on.

Take a Breather

Because stretching out your meal over 20 minutes can be challenging at first, you can chew your food until it's liquefied, or you can take small breaks. Try pausing briefly after every few bites or drink a little water during the breaks.

Get Rid of Distractions

Eating while watching TV or working is one of the causes of mindless eating. Because your focus is split between your meal and the other activity, you might not be mindful of the pace at which you are eating. So consider mealtime your singular focus.

Enjoy the Flavor

A useful principle to apply when learning how to eat slowly is to eat for taste and enjoyment. Be mindful of the flavor in each bite and savor your meal. Savoring food not only saves you calories but can also teach you how to appreciate the taste of good food as well. Meditate on your food, its smell, texture, and taste.

---

82 McDonald, A. (2010, October 19). Why eating slowly may help you feel full faster. *Harvard Health Publications.* Retrieved from http://www.health.harvard.edu/blog/why-eating-slowly-may-help-you-feel-full-faster-20101019605

CHAPTER 49

LEARN FROM SLIPS

E veryone wants to get weight loss perfect the first time round. For most humans, it is a journey of trial and error. Every mistake, though, can lead to a better understanding of how to be successful at weight loss. If you beat yourself up or allow yourself to feel defeated, there is a good chance you will give up entirely. So instead of becoming discouraged when you slip, see it as the learning opportunity it is. Ask yourself what can you learn from the experience? What can you do differently next time? Do you need any additional resources? Who or what can help you? Remember, each meal is opportunity for success and each day is an opportunity to start new and fresh. When it comes to healthy eating and weight loss, it is what you do 90% of the time that counts, not the 10%.

Here are some of the most popular slips people make with weight loss:

Doing Too Much Too Fast

It's only natural to want to do everything you can to shed weight. However, doing too much too soon can actually be detrimental to your efforts. Losing weight and keeping it off is about adopting healthy habits at a steady pace. If you rush the process, you'll only end up where you started.

Choosing the Wrong Diet

A pitfall that is all too common is choosing a fad diet that promises dramatic results in a short time. While it may be possible to lose a lot of weight quickly, it is not possible to maintain it over the long run; people usually just gain the weight back and sometimes more! Look for and choose diets that promote healthy weight loss of 1-2 lbs. each week instead.

Underestimating Food Portions

Many people who want to lose weight underestimate food portions and sabotage weight loss by eating more than they think.[83] If you are used to eating out of large plates, try a smaller plate size instead.

Miscounting Calories

Calorie-counting can be tricky for both beginners and the experienced alike. Like any skill, it needs to be practiced and mastered over time. If you tend to over- or underestimate your daily intake, refine your food label reading skills and use a log to keep track of what you eat.

Exercising Too Much

Working out several times a week can fast-track weight loss. However, overtraining can derail your efforts by causing injury and even compromising your immune system. If you're recovering from an injury or caught the flu, use this slip to adjust your fitness routine. It also helps to lower the intensity. If you are just getting started with a new exercise program, go slowly and establish a safe foundation. Sore muscles and injuries are not going to motivate you!

Setting an Unrealistic Goal

Aspiring to look like you did in your teen years when you are 50 years old or expecting to have a body of a smaller-framed person is not a winning formula. Take your age, gender, height, frame, activity level, and overall health into account when developing you weight-loss goals.

---

83   Ledikwe, J. H., Ello-Martin, J. A., & Rolls, B. J. (2005). Portion sizes and the obesity epidemic. *The Journal of Nutrition 135*(4), 905-909. Retrieved from http://jn.nutrition.org/content/135/4/905.long

CHAPTER 50

DON'T SHOW UP HUNGRY

E vents and gatherings can be tricky if you are trying to lose weight. They are filled with people, music, and, of course, lots of delicious food. While you might think it's a good idea to skip a meal and eat at the event to avoid calories, it will end up working against your calorie intake and you are likely to eat way more than if you didn't' skip the meal. Here's why:

Skipping a meal and allowing yourself to starve for a while can cause you to overeat when you finally have your meal. People tend to eat faster and choose larger portions when they're famished. Eating faster means your brain won't have time to register fullness, and bigger portions carry more calories.

Also, there is scientific research that suggests people eat more in social settings than at home. Music, dim lighting, and social influence have been associated with overeating.[84] And because you have skipped a meal, you think you are "entitled" to eat whatever you want, but your body can only process so many calories at once before it wants to store the excess as fat.

Bottom line: don't show up hungry. At the very least, have a light snack before you leave for the event. Choose snack foods that are low in calories and high in protein and fiber, which can help you feel satisfied in just a few bites (e.g., a cup of soup, an apple with a little peanut butter, half a turkey sandwich on whole grain bread).

If it's too late to grab a healthy snack at home, here are some strategies you can use to choose smarter at the dinner table:

Drink Water

Have a glass of water before dinner or take sips while eating so you feel full earlier. If you're still hungry after the meal, have another glass and wait 15 minutes before going for seconds.

Eat Slowly

You can resist overeating by chewing your food slowly. Take your time with every mouthful and savor the flavor of the meal.

Dish up on Smaller Plates

Serving meals on small plates is a good strategy for controlling portions and calories. Go for flat, open dishware and avoid bowls.

Fill Your Plate with Veggies

You can still salvage your calorie budget by choosing what goes on your plate. Cut back calories by filling most of your plate with salads and greens. Add moderate amounts of protein to make the meal more satisfying. Watch out for the heavy sauces, salad dressings, and simple carbohydrates!

---

84 Wansink, B. (2004). Environmental factors that increase the food intake and consumption volume of unknowing consumers. *Annual Reviews 11*(7). Retrieved from http://foodpsychology.cornell.edu/sites/default/files/Consumption-ARN_2004.pdf

CHAPTER 51

WORST FOODS FOR WEIGHT LOSS

While the title of this book is about losing weight without giving up the foods you love, which is absolutely true, it is important to realize that some foods will actually do the opposite— put on the pounds and affect your health in a negative way. If you are serious about losing weight, then you need to avoid or limit the following foods in your diet:

Diet Soda

Marketed as a refreshing beverage that gives you the taste of soda without the calories, diet soda is not a dieter's friend. In fact, just the opposite, research studies are associating diet soda with weight gain.

Diet sodas contain certain artificial sweeteners that the body mistakes for regular sugar. When these sweeteners enter your system, your body releases insulin to help break the sugars down as normal. Because the sugars are artificial and not real, you end up with high levels of insulin which ultimately causes weight gain.[85]

A study in *Behavioral Neuroscience* also suggests that the sweet taste of soda increases appetite.[86] Adult male rats fed sweeteners regularly ate more calories daily and showed a significant increase in body weight.

White Flour Foods

From baked goods and pasta to cereals, foods made with white flours are a recipe for weight gain.[87] With little fiber and lots of refined carbohydrates, these foods offer little nutritional value and many empty calories. Additionally, these foods contain simple carbohydrates, which means that they release a lot of sugar into your blood stream. Your body can't handle it and ends up converting the sugar to fat. And because these foods are processed quickly in your digestive system, you become hungry sooner.

Trans Fats Foods

Fat is generally divided into saturated and unsaturated types, but there is a third, more sinister type called trans fats. These fats can appear in food naturally, usually in very small amounts or can be added to foods artificially or through frying with hydrogenated oils. They are used to extend shelf life and add to texture and taste.

Unfortunately though, this type of fat is a major contributor to heart disease, stroke, and type 2 diabetes. Consuming trans fats also has negative effects on weight loss because it redistributes throughout the body, often leading to fat tissue gathering in the belly area, hindering the liver from burning fats efficiently.[88]

High Fructose Corn Syrup

High fructose corn syrup (HFCS) is corn syrup whose glucose has been partially changed into a different sugar, fructose. It is not a naturally occurring food product, but one that has been created by manufacturers.

High-fructose corn syrup is much cheaper than table sugar to make and can taste sweeter too, which is a problem because if you get used to the sweetness of HFCS, you will find naturally sweet foods not so sweet! You will find it in soft drinks, baked goods, sauces, dairy products—almost everywhere!

Manufacturers claim that it makes food taste better and improves texture. However, there is a strong correlation between the use of HFCS and obesity, increase in body fat metabolic problems, diabetes, and a weakened immune system.[89, 90]

Be sure to read labels and avoid HFCS as well as products with a lot of sugar both for your overall health as well as for losing weight.

Salty Foods

Over the years, health organizations have noticed an alarming trend that could be fuelling the obesity problem: the high intake of salt. Despite the recommended intake of 1,500 milligrams, most Americans far exceed this limit daily, increasing the risk of weight gain and other health issues.[91]

Salt in itself might not be fattening, but it can trigger chemical reactions that shift your bathroom scale in the wrong direction. When you consume more salt than needed, it can overpower your kidneys and send sodium back into your bloodstream.

With too much salt in your system, your body is susceptible to retaining water. This leads to water retention (water weight) and bloating. You can pack on a few pounds in a short amount of time. By simply cutting back on salt, the water can be flushed out and leave you slimmer with little effort.

---

85 Suez, J., Korem, T., Zeevi, D., Zilberman-Schapira, G., Thaiss, C. A., Maza, O.... Elinav, E. (2014). Artificial sweeteners induce glucose intolerance by altering gut microbiota. *Nature*, *5*(14), 181-186. Retrieved from http://www.nature.com/nature/journal/v514/n7521/full/nature13793.html

86 Swithers, S. E., & Davidson, D. L. (2008). The role of sweet taste: Calorie predictive relations in energy regulation by rats. *Behavioral Neuroscience*, *122*(1), 161-173. Retrieved from http://www.ncbi.nlm.nih.gov/pubmed/?term=A+Role+for+Sweet+Taste%3A+Calorie+Predictive+Relations+in+Energy+Regulation

87 Hu, F. B. (2010). Are refined carbohydrates worse than saturated fat? *The American Journal of Clinical Nutrition*, *91*(6), 1541-1542. Retrieved from http://ajcn.nutrition.org/content/91/6/1541.short

88 Bendsen, N. T., Chabanova, E., Thomsen, H. S., Larsen, T. M., Newman, J.W., Stender, S.,... Astrup, A. (2011). Effect of trans fatty acid intake on abdominal and liver fat deposition and blood lipids: A randomized trial in overweight postmenopausal women. *Nutrition and Diabetes 1*, e4. Retrieved from http://www.nature.com/nutd/journal/v1/n1/full/nutd20104a.html

89 Mercola, J. (n.d.). High-fructose corn syrup. Retrieved from http://www.mercola.com/ebook/high-fructose-corn-syrup.aspx

90 Princeton University. (2010, March 22). High-fructose corn syrup prompts considerably more weight gain, researchers find. *ScienceDaily*. Retrieved from http://www.sciencedaily.com/releases/2010/03/100322121115.htm

91 Reinberg, S. (2013). Americans still eat too much salt: CDC. *Health Day*. Retrieved from http://consumer.healthday.com/public-health-information-30/centers-for-disease-control-news-120/americans-still-eat-too-much-salt-cdc-683236.html

ADDITIONAL PUBLICATIONS OF INTEREST

ABS! 50 OF THE BEST CORE EXERCISES TO STRENGTHEN, TONE, AND FLATTEN YOUR BELLY.

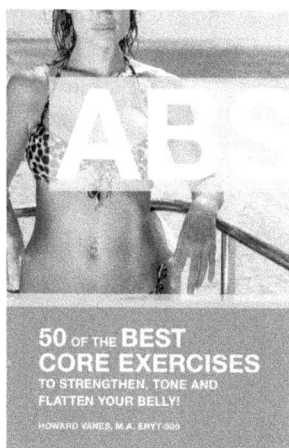

Experience 50 of the very best ab and stomach exercises from Yoga, Pilates and other fitness modalities. They have been carefully selected for their ability to produce quick results and are fun to do. ABS! Goes well beyond old-fashioned crunches and sit-ups so you can have an extremely effective abs workout.

Whether your belly is on the soft side or you're a high-level athlete, you'll find a great variety of ab exercises, which will target all four major groups of abdominal muscles, categorized by easy, moderate and challenging—so it is great for all levels of fitness.

This book doesn't make extreme promises like getting ripped abs in 6 days, doesn't recommend crazy diets that you're dying to get off of in a week, and there isn't a lot of technical mumbo-jumbo! When you purchase this book, you will get highly effective ab and stomach exercises that will help you strengthen, tone, and get a flat belly—in a healthy way.

Chapters include: 50 of the best exercises for your abs with photos and clear instructions, discussion of the many benefits of core exercises, overview of anatomy and more!

THE BRAIN FITNESS AND BETTER MEMORY BOOK

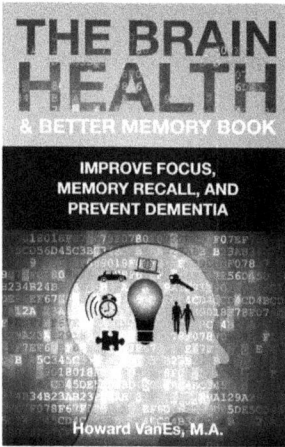

Most of us will experience some type of decline in mental sharpness, focus, and memory as we age. This can result in any number of problems, including forgetfulness, moodiness, insomnia, lack of problem-solving skills, and an inability to communicate effectively.

When brain health deterioration becomes more severe, it can lead to dementia and the problems associated with it including confusion, difficultly understanding visual images, changes in personality, trouble remembering, hallucinations, and lack of judgment.

Your brain plays a major role in almost everything you do, including thinking, feeling, communicating, breathing, remembering, working, playing, sleeping, etc. Vital to the quality of your life, therefore, is maintaining or improving the health of your brain.

This book will identify the issues that cause a reduction in brain fitness and memory, explaining how each impacts your brain and then offer ideas, tips, and tools to optimize the health of your brain.

Order a copy of this book today and start your journey to a healthier brain and better memory!

YOGA: THE BACK PAIN CURE

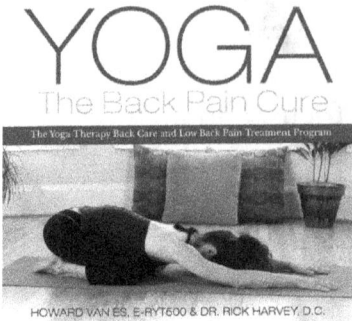

YOGA
The Back Pain Cure
The Yoga Therapy Back Care and Low Back Pain Treatment Program

HOWARD VAN ES, E-RYT500 & DR. RICK HARVEY, D.C.

Back pain! As anyone with a backache will tell you, pain, limited activities, and days missed from work take their toll physically, financially, and emotionally.

A big problem with most back-care programs is limited treatment options. Pain medications often mask problems, allowing further damage to occur because warning pain is not felt. Physical therapy is limited by what insurance companies deem necessary, and, lastly, surgery, a costly option, is often ineffective.

The good news is that yoga therapy can help relieve your pain while at the same time improve flexibility and strength. This book features two yoga therapy practices. The first is for acute back problems, which means you're in pain right now. This practice is designed to bring structural balance back into your body and gently stretch key muscles, reducing pain and helping you heal. The second practice is designed to build strength and flexibility, which helps prevent future problems.

With the help of this book, you can get back into the activities and lifestyle you enjoy, without drugs or costly treatments, and in the comfort of your home.

RELEASE YOUR SHOULDERS, RELAX YOUR NECK: THE BEST EXERCISES FOR RELIEVING SHOULDER TENSION AND NECK PAIN.

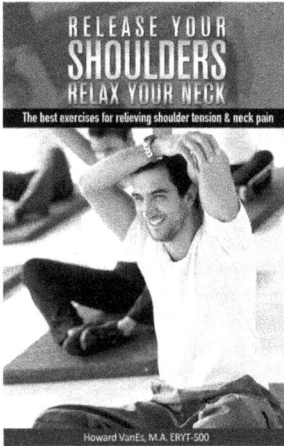

Do you suffer from shoulder pain or shoulder tension? How about neck pain?

In this book discover:

- **The main causes of shoulder and neck pain.**
- **How to eliminate shoulder tension and neck pain with 53 highly effective shoulder and neck exercises.**
- **Photos of the exercises with easy to follow instructions.**
- **Key prevention strategies to stop problems before they start so you can have healthy shoulders and a pain-free neck.**
- **Why computer users are at high risk for injury and what to do to significantly reduce your risk.**
- **Anatomy of the shoulder joints, how they move and why they can get so tight.**

This book is a must for people who work on computers, dental hygienists, hair stylists, athletes and anyone who carries a lot of stress in their neck or shoulders.

INSOMNIA: HOW CAN I GET TO SLEEP?

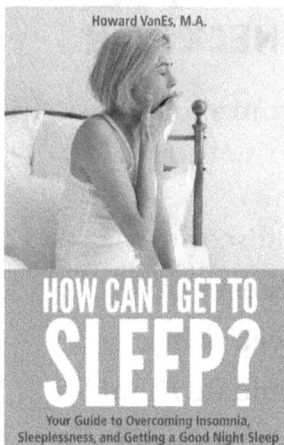

Howard VanEs, M.A.

HOW CAN I GET TO SLEEP?

Your Guide to Overcoming Insomnia, Sleeplessness, and Getting a Good Night Sleep

If you have you had trouble sleeping, you are in very good company, as 58% of adults experience insomnia regularly. Lying awake, tossing and turning, mental agitations and the exhaustion that follows are definitely not any fun!

The side effects of insomnia can reduce your productivity, make you irritable, and lead to numerous physical ailments, including obesity, hypertension, lack of coordination, weight gain, etc.

In this book you'll:

- **Discover what is really keeping you up at night; the answer might surprise you!**
- **The best non-drug methods for getting to sleep naturally with our "Insomnia Tool Box."**
- **How to get back to sleep when you wake up in the middle of the night.**
- **Reduce and eliminate tension and anxiety with powerful techniques that help quiet your mind, remove stress from your body, and slip easily into a good night's sleep.**
- **How to eat your way to a good night sleep: which foods actually help you fall asleep and which will keep you from falling asleep.**

ABOUT THE AUTHOR

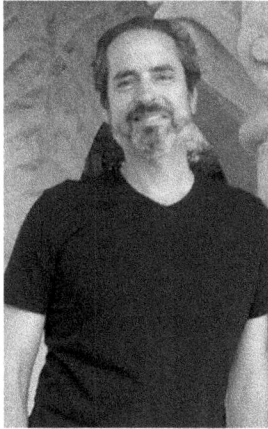

Howard VanEs, M.A., E-RYT 500 has been committed to wellness and fitness for over 30 years. He has a deep passion for helping people learn about the many ways they can improve the quality of their health and empower their lives through natural methods of healing.

Howard has written over 20 books, most focused on health and wellness. Many of his books have been best sellers in their respective categories on Amazon. For over 24 years, Howard has been a dedicated practitioner of hatha yoga, and has been teaching yoga for the last 19 years in the Bay Area of California. Howard also has a M.A. in counseling psychology and is a former psychotherapist.

You can learn more about Howard and his books at www. BooksonHealth.net

www.ingramcontent.com/pod-product-compliance
Lightning Source LLC
Chambersburg PA
CBHW072138270326
41931CB00010B/1795